Clinical Pearls in Diagnostic Cardiac Computed Tomographic Angiography

Muzammil H. Musani • Eric J. Feldmann
Michael Poon

Clinical Pearls in Diagnostic Cardiac Computed Tomographic Angiography

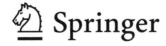

Muzammil H. Musani
Department of Medicine and Radiology
Stony Brook University Hospital
Stony Brook, NY
USA

Eric J. Feldmann
Department of Radiology
Stony Brook University Hospital
Stony Brook, NY
USA

Michael Poon
Department of Medicine and Radiology
Stony Brook University Hospital
Stony Brook, NY
USA

ISBN 978-3-319-08167-0   ISBN 978-3-319-08168-7   (eBook)
DOI 10.1007/978-3-319-08168-7

Library of Congress Control Number: 2015943704

Springer Cham Heidelberg New York Dordrecht London
© Springer International Publishing Switzerland 2015

Printed on acid-free paper

Springer International Publishing AG Switzerland is part of Springer Science+Business Media (www.springer.com)

Preface

Clinical Pearls in Diagnostic Cardiac Computed Tomographic Angiography is a compilation of some of the most thought-provoking cases in cardiovascular imaging using CT. This concise book is specifically designed as a beginner's tool to lay the foundation for residents, fellows and physicians who have interest in cardiovascular CT. Those who are studying for licensure exam will find the cases and discussions in this book to be extremely beneficial. In our experience, practitioners must not only know how to interpret cardiac CTA, but also understand the basic principles of scanning in order to master the field of cardiac imaging. Therefore, we have placed strong emphasis on simplifying basic physics principles and applying them to daily scanning routines. We provide interpretation of challenging cases in various aspects of cardiac imaging, such as coronary artery disease, anomalous coronary arteries, congenital heart disease, coronary artery bypass grafts, infectious diseases, structural heart disease, tumors, and aortic pathology. All images are high resolution reproductions with subsequent cardiac catheterization imaging for cases where obstructive coronary artery disease was revealed.

Stony Brook, NY, USA   Muzammil H. Musani, MD

Acknowledgements

To my parents Muhammad Hanif and Kulsoom Hanif for their tremendous sacrifices and encouragement.

To my wife Ayesha for putting up with long hours during my fellowship training and our children Daanya, Muhammad and Nusaybah for bringing unexplainable joy and happiness. I would like to thank my siblings Sadaf and Anis for putting up with my childhood. To Dr. and Mrs. Master for their unrelenting support.

I would like to express my gratitude to my mentors during residency, cardiac imaging and cardiology fellowships. Finally, would like to thank all the contributing authors and radiology staff at Stony Brook University Hospital.

Muzammil H. Musani, MD

Contents

Introduction to Cardiac Computed Tomography

Muzammil H. Musani and Eric J. Feldmann

Recent dramatic technological advances in computed tomography (CT) technology allow routine performance of cardiac computed tomography angiography (CCTA) with excellent image quality at modest effective radiation doses (E). Improved z-axis coverage, utilizing scanners with 64, 128, 256, and 320 z-axis detector-rows, decreases "slab artifact," improves contrast opacification, and allows shorter breath holds – thus further decreasing cardiac motion artifacts and improving overall image quality. Improved "true" hardware-dependent temporal resolution, now at roughly 100–175 ms with single source and 75 ms with dual source scanners, decreases artifacts from coronary artery motion. Improved detector technology now yields a maximal spatial resolution on the order of 18.2 line pairs/cm.

CCTA has truly transformed from the exotic to the routine in the last decade. This chapter focuses on the underlying principles pivotal in this transformation: basic CCTA physics, patient preparation, image acquisition, imaging techniques/protocols, postprocessing techniques, and artifacts/artifact reduction.

1.1 CT Scanner Basics

The main components of a CT scanner are the gantry (containing the detector row/photon source unit), table, and the computer software/hardware to process the raw data. The gantry is donut-shaped and contains a photon source opposite a panel of detectors that both rotate around the patient/table in the x-y plane as a fixed unit opposite each other (Fig. 1.1). Dual source scanners have two such units at roughly 90° offset in the x-y plane. Typically the speed of this rotation ranges from 0.2 to 0.35 s/rev in most modern scanners and is the most important determinant of true temporal resolution in CT, which is calculated as half the time for a full rotation plus an angular correction for the fan beam geometry (Fig. 1.2). This yields temporal resolutions of roughly 100–175 ms with single source and 75 ms with dual source scanners. The source detector unit is continuously moving throughout the entire exam; however the delivery of photons can be turned off and on quite rapidly, as well as the mA (amount of photons) adjusted (e.g., automatic tube current modulation and EKG gated tube current modulation). Although slower, the kVp can also be changed to different energies on dual energy scanners.

Similar to MRI, when describing a CT scanner, it is customary to consider the long-axis of the table the z-axis, and the short axis the x-y plane. The photon source is a point source, in that it creates an Elliptical cone of photons from a focal spot. The angle of the elliptical cone in the x-y plane is called fan angle, and in the z-plane is called cone angle. Fan angle is typically around 40–50° and determines the maximum x-y plane of image reconstruction or scan field of view (SFOV) of the study. Manufacturers typically allow you to choose SFOV (sometimes called

M.H. Musani et al., *Clinical Pearls in Diagnostic Cardiac Computed Tomographic Angiography*, DOI 10.1007/978-3-319-08168-7_1, © Springer International Publishing Switzerland 2015

Fig. 1.1 Gantry with radiation tube (photon source) and detector rows, also depicting cone beam angle and fan angle (Picture Courtesy of Michael Poon MD)

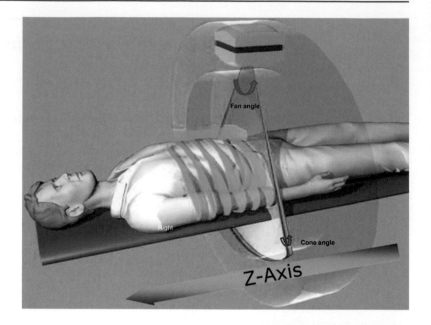

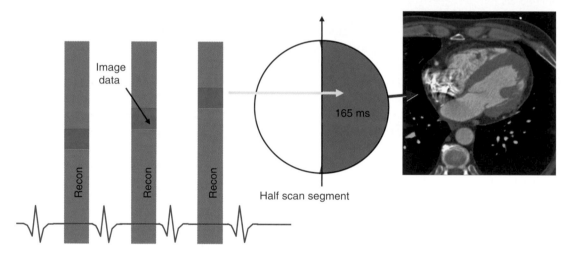

Fig. 1.2 Reconstruction of an image using data from half gantry rotation. To create an axial image, we only require an approximate data from half of the scan rotation plus fan angle. This then gives us a an approximate temporal reso-lution of 165 ms based on a gantry rotation of 330 ms. The orange boxes are image data reconstructed at the same phase of the cardiac cycle (Picture Courtesy of Michael Poon MD)

calibrated field of view) for a scan. Ranges vary from 18 to 50 cm. For CCTA, typically 320–400 mm is used as this covers the majority of patient x-y axis size. Cone angle is very small with 64 detector row CT scanners, but become substantially larger with the use of 256×0.625mm or 320×0.5 mm collimation. Cone angle and the number of detectors in the z-axis determine the amount of z-axis coverage acquired with one gantry rotation (Fig. 1.3) [1].

There are a few scanning techniques available on current CT scanners. A scout tomogram is obtained without rotation of the gantry, just with table movement and a few detector rows. The image has an appearance grossly similar to a standard AP, PA, or lateral radiograph. It is per-formed on all exams to plot the z-axis and x-y plane coverage needed. Once the gantry is spin-ning, two acquisition methods are available, depending on whether or not the table is moving

Fig. 1.3 Simplified representation of cone beam angle and fan angle. Typically there are several hundred detectors which are concave towards the radiation source. For a 64-detector row scanner, cone and fan angles are usually around 2.4 and 60 degrees, respectively

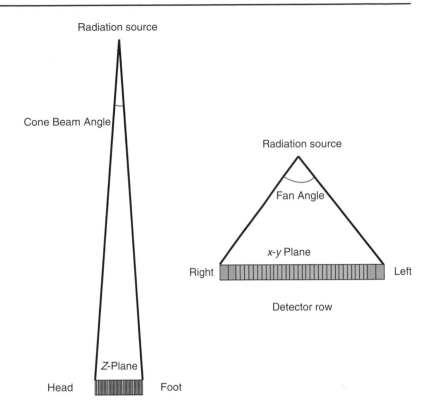

during scanning. If the table is moving during image acquisition then it is called "helical" or "spiral" acquisition. If the table is not moving during imaging acquisition then it is called "step and shoot," "sequential," "axial," or "volume scanning." Currently (except for in dual-source scanners), the prospectively triggered "step and shoot" acquisition is preferred in most routine applications of CCTA [2].

1.2   Resolution

1.2.1   Temporal Resolution

Temporal resolution is simply defined as the shortest acquisition time necessary to reconstruct an image. It is analogous to the shutter speed of your camera. It can be thought of as having hardware (gantry rotation speed in rev/msec) and software (i.e., multisegment reconstruction, half scan reconstruction) components. Further discussion on its effect on image quality is elaborated in the coronary motion artifact section.

1.2.2   Spatial Resolution (High Contrast Resolution)

The ability to discern the edges between adjacent small objects that differ greatly in attenuation. It is typically thought of as intrinsic to a scanner and defined by a bar phantom (in line pairs per centimeter). Although, there are also postprocessing/reconstruction methods that may increase apparent spatial resolution (sharper kernel, overlapping slices, etc.). It is defined in both in the x-y and z planes. It corresponds to typical voxel/pixel values of around 0.3–0.6 mm on today's scanners. Spatial resolution is crucial in coronary CTA because the contrast filled coronary artery lumen (250–500 HU) demonstrates high contrast with the background of epicardial fat (−30 to −100 HU).

1.2.3   Contrast Resolution (Low Contrast Resolution)

The ability to distinguish between objects of similar attenuation; for example a 10 HU liver lesion in the background of 50 HU liver paren-chyma. It is typically dependent on image sig-nal to noise ratio and is quantitatively defined by a low-contrast phantom for a given tech-nique/scanner. For enhancing structures on contrast enhanced exams, it may be improved utilizing lower kV (80–100 kVp) technique. Typically, low contrast resolution is not as important in coronary CTA as spatial resolution because the contrast filled coronary artery lumen (250–500 HU) demonstrates high con-trast with the background of epicardial fat (−30 to −100 HU). It is more relevant in CT myocar-dial perfusion imaging.

1.3   Basic Principles of CCTA Image Acquisition

CCTA fundamentally differs from most routine CTs in that on top of it being respiratory gated (utilizing a breath hold) – it is EKG gated. EKG gating simply means synchronizing CT data acquisition to a specific cardiac "phase." Phase is defined as a percentage of the R-R interval, so that for a person with a heart rate of 60 bpm 30 % would be near end systole and 75 % would be near end diastole. Although it is arbitrary, it is a more specific nomenclature than the traditional phases of the cardiac cycle taught in physiology. There are two modes of ECG synchronized acquisition:
1. Prospective ECG triggering
2. Retrospective ECG gating

1.3.1   Prospective ECG Triggering with Step and Shoot Technique

This is a technique where the previous few heart beat R-R intervals are used to predict the expected future R-R interval. Typically this is utilized with step and shoot scanning. The data are only col-lected at a predefined phase (typically 750 ms at 60 bpm), and for a predefined time interval (mini-mum 350 ms at 60 bpm), which is determined by a user defined delay before acquisition (Fig. 1.4). Depending on the scanner z-axis collimation per rotation, the step and shoot will continue until the scanning is completed in the z-axis. For example, if the region of interest (heart) being scanned is 16 cm, for a 64 detector-row single source scan-ner with 0.625 mm detectors (4 cm coverage dur-ing a single gantry rotation), it will take 4 scans or "steps" to cover the z-axis of the entire heart (Fig. 1.5) . Vis-a-vis a 320 detector-row scanner with a maximum of 16 cm z-axis coverage per rotation will acquire the entire z-axis of the heart in one scan (Fig. 1.6).

1.3.2   Retrospective ECG Gating and Helical Acquisition

In this technique, beginning essentially at any point in the cardiac cycle, the patient is moved through the gantry during continuous scanning. The pitch is typically 0.2–0.3 during retrospec-tive scanning, which yields a typical scan time of 7–9 heartbeats. During image postprocessing,

Fig. 1.4 *Blue line* indicates the five heart beats (R-R intervals) used to predict the R-R interval at the time of image acquisition *yellow line*. *Light gray* area represents the segment of R-R interval acquired during scanning

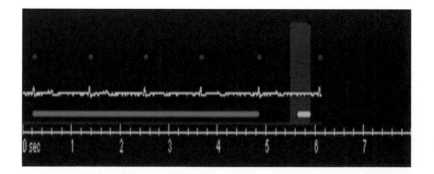

Fig. 1.5 ECG gated prospectively triggered (or "step and shoot" sequential) scanning on a 64-detector row CT scanner (Picture Courtesy of Michael Poon MD)

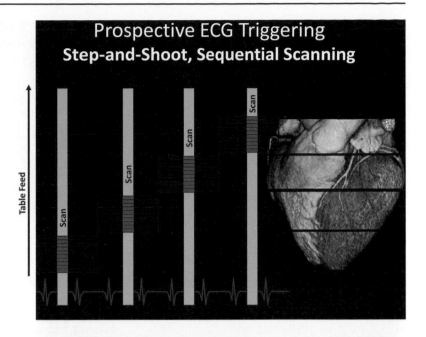

Fig. 1.6 ECG gated prospective triggered scanning on a 320-detector row scanner

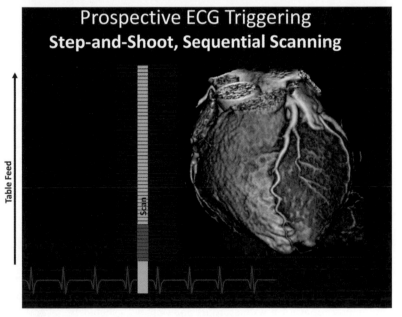

cardiac phases are assigned "in retrospect" using ECG to source images, occasionally with multi-segment reconstruction (Fig. 1.7).

Pitch is a term only used in helical imaging, and is a unitless ratio defined as:

Pitch = Table feed in one 360° rotation (mm)/Total collimated slice width (mm)

Retrospective ECG gating in single source scanners has fallen out of favor due to the high radiation burden. It is typically reserved for patients with high heart rates, arrhythmia, or where systolic images are necessary. However, prospectively triggered high-pitch helical acquisition in dual-source scanners with a pitch

Fig. 1.7 Retrospective
ECG-gated CT scanning
(Picture Courtesy of
Michael Poon MD)

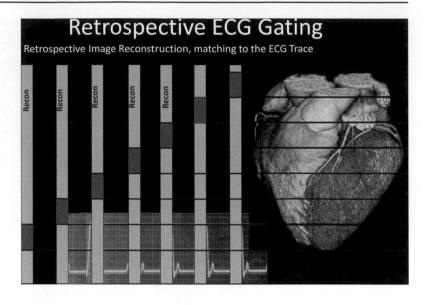

of 3.4 may be performed with exceptionally
low radiation dose and an approximate temporal resolution of 75 ms.

1.3.3   Patient Preparation

Patient preparation is crucial for good quality
images. There are white papers on this topic read-
ily available from the large societies.

The patient should be consented and have
recent lab work including BUN/creatine and
beta HCG as warranted. Patients must be
screened for any contraindication to contrast agent (allergy, renal insufficiency), beta
blocker (chronic obstructive pulmonary disease, allergy), and nitroglycerine (severe aortic stenosis, recent use of phosphodiesterase
inhibitors, etc.). Patients with contrast allergy
may need preparation with steroids and benad-
ryl. Radiation dose concerns are also addressed
at this time.

A medium to large bore (16-20 G) peripheral
intravenous line is placed, preferably in the ante-
cubital fossa of the right arm. Central lines may
also be utilized, assuming the tip is in the superior vena cava or right atrium and they are
approved for high injection rates and pressure
injector.

Patients with a heart rate of >65 bpm depending on the technology should be premedicated
with oral beta blockers, typically 50–100 mg
metoprolol depending on heart rate about one
hour prior to the scanning procedure. Patient can
also be medicated at the scanner using IV metoprolol (typically 5 mg IV push and may repeat
injection in 2 min intervals up to three to five
times), while continuously monitoring vital
signs. Calcium channel blockers are reserved for
patients where beta blockers are contraindicated
(0.25 mg/kg IV, or 20 mg for an average patient,
as a bolus administered over 2 min) [3].

1.3.4   Scanning the Patient

Typically, the patient is placed on the CT scanner
table in the supine position, with feet first. Care
should be taken to remove all metallic ornaments
from the body prior to scanning. ECG lead wires
should be moved to the side and should be left on the
chest. A sublingual nitroglycerin tab (typically
0.4 mcg) is given to the patient about 3–5 min before
the exam, as long as no contraindications exist.

1.3.4.1 Scouts
Postero-anterior (PA) and lateral views for plot-
ting z-axis and SFOV are performed (Fig. 1.8).

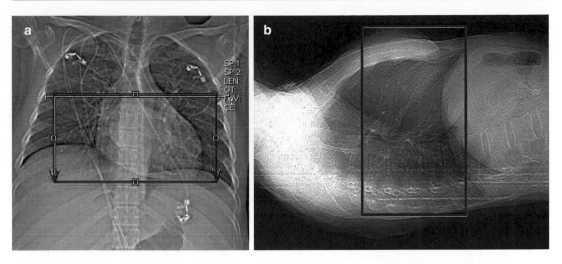

Fig. 1.8 Antero-posterior (panel **a**) and lateral (panel **b**) scout images are used to define the scan field of view

1.3.5 Noncontrast for Coronary Artery Calcium Scoring (CACS)

In most patients, a noncontrast cardiac CT is performed at 120 kV with variable mAs based on body habitus, specifically for calcium scoring. It typically adds between 40 and 80 mGy×cm of DLP to the exam. CACS is performed for a few reasons:

1. For CAD risk stratification based on the extensive literature and population health studies (e.g., MESA) on the association between the severity of coronary calcium burden and the extent of coronary artery disease.
2. By evaluating the noncontrast image, the technologist can more accurately prescribe the z-axis for the CCTA. Since the technique for CCTA is typically higher radiation than CACS, this may result in radiation dose equalization or savings.
3. Allows quantitative evaluation of coronary artery calcium burden (e.g., Agatston's method, volume score, distribution specific score, vessel specific score, lesion specific score, etc.). This is useful for risk factor stratification in certain patients.
4. Allows differentiation of coronary wall calcium from contrast filled lumen by visually referencing/subtracting the two studies.

Occasionally calcium and contrast will have the same HU and may be difficult or impossible to differentiate.

5. Allows more thoughtful CCTA technique alterations such as kV, mAs, and the degree of padding necessary. Padding is defined as scanning a given z-axis slice for more time than the minimum amount necessary to reconstruct an image. It is commonly performed to acquire a greater percentage of the R-R interval as a hedge in patients with higher heart rates and those with R-R interval variability.
6. Sometimes exams will be changed or canceled based on the findings from the CACS (e.g., stents present, excessive calcium burden, coronary motion artifact, etc.).

1.3.6 Cardiac CTA Scan

The scan is performed utilizing 30–100 ml of typically 300–370 mg/ml nonionic injected at a rate of 4–5 ml/s. Parameters such as kVp, mAs, rotation time, prospective vs retrospective technique, need for delayed imaging, z-axis coverage, multisegment reconstruction, and %R-R interval to scan are set by the imaging specialist prior to the exam.

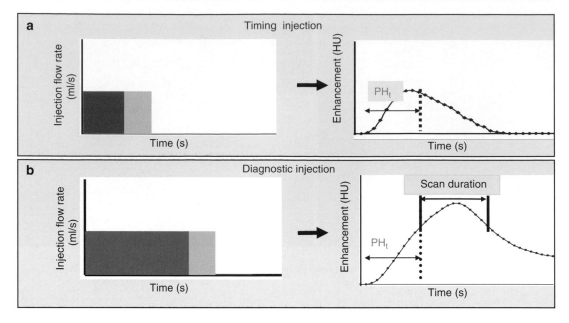

Fig. 1.9 Timing bolus: Panel (**a**) Test bolus injection of about 20 ml of contrast followed by another 15 ml of saline. Panel (**b**) Diagnostic injection of 50–100 ml of contrast followed by 50 ml of saline using the same injection rate as that of the test bolus (Picture Courtesy of Michael Poon MD)

1.3.7 Contrast Administration

Two modes of contrast administration are:
1. Timing bolus
2. Bolus tracking
   a) Automatic triggering
   b) Manual triggering

1.3.7.1 Timing Bolus
Before the scan, an injection of 15–20 ml of contrast agent is performed while continuously scanning a single slice in the descending aorta, generating a time-enhancement curve. The time of peak enhancement plus a scanner dependent fudge factor (Typically of 5 or more seconds) is used as the time delay prior to the actual contrast enhanced scan (Fig. 1.9).

1.3.7.2 Bolus Tracking
During bolus tracking, the entire volume of contrast is administered at a rate of typically 4–5 ml/s while continuously scanning at a single slice level in the descending aorta, thus generating time-enhancement curve in real-time. Once a predetermined HU level is reached, the scan is started (either automatically or manually depending on software/preference (Fig. 1.10). A lower dose of IV contrast is utilized in bolus tracking as there is no need for the extra 15–20 ml needed to perform a timing bolus. A drawback of bolus tracking is that it depends on an region of interest (ROI). Occasionally scans may be started prematurely or late due to abundant adjacent calcification, patient motion, and/or other artifacts that resulted in inaccurate HU measurements.

1.4 Cardiac CT Imaging Postprocessing

1.4.1 Image Display

Typical display matrices and field of view (DFOV) are 512×512 and around 240 mm. This is because each pixel size (240 mm/512=0.47 mm) closely matches the maximum inherent spatial resolution of today's scanners (around 0.4–0.6 mm). Wider DFOV may be performed to evaluate peripheral structures, up to the scan field of view (SFOV). DFOV is always equal to or less than the SFOV. Typical SFOV are 320–400 mm depending on patient size and exam ordered. With continued advances in spatial resolution 1,024×1,024 reconstruction matrices may become the norm. Window width and center are typically manipulated in real time to provide contrast between certain structures as needed and is not a "fixed" phenomenon.

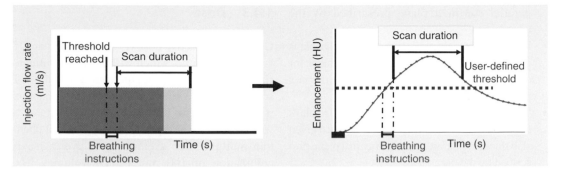

Fig. 1.10 Bolus monitoring or tracking: A large bolus of contrast followed by another smaller bolus of saline are being injected by a power injector as shown on the *left panel*. The contrast intensity is being tracked continu- ously until it reaches a predetermined level of Hounsfield units (the *red dotted straight line*) as shown on the *right panel* and the scanning process is initiated (the *black dou- ble headed arrow*)

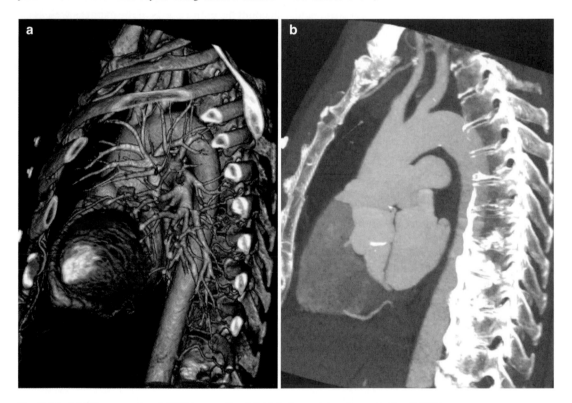

Fig. 1.11   (a) Volume rendered (VR) image. Panel (**b**) Maximum intensity projection (MIP) image

CCTA interpretation typically requires advanced software that possesses capabilities above and beyond those of a traditional picture archive and communication system (PACS) – although this dynamic is in constant flux. There are numerous products available, all of which have the ability for advanced postprocessing and dis- play, and typically have dedicated hardware/server for this purpose, as the datasets can reach 10,000 images (5 GB) and sometimes need to be dis- played instantaneously via a cine loop.

Postprocessing techniques include:
- Axial (source images): the starting point of all postprocessing techniques
- Volume rendered images: The user defines thresholds for opacity, color, and brightness for a given HU in an isovolumetric dataset and dis- plays the image as a three-dimensional struc- ture Fig. 1.11.
- Maximum intensity projection (MIP): Displays only the voxels with maximum HU number for a given slab thickness along a

parallel ray in a plane prescribed by the user.

- Minimum intensity projection (minIP): Displays only the voxels with minimum HU number for a given slab thickness along a parallel ray in a plane prescribed by the user.
- Thick multiplanar reformation (MPR): Displays the average HU number of voxels within a given slab thickness along a parallel ray in a plane prescribed by the user.
- Orthogonal multiplanar reformation: Routine sagittal and coronal reformations in the orthogonal planes of the CT table/gantry.
- Oblique multiplanar reformations: With iso-volumetric datasets (where voxel size, and this displayed pixel size, is the same in the x-y and z-axes) any angle/projection may be displayed with the same resolution as the native axial plane. This allows traditional cardiac planes to be prescribed, as well as curved (cMPR) and straightened (sMPR) reformations to be prescribed along numerous planes along a curved structure.

1.4.2   Interpretation

The mainstay of CCTA interpretation is oblique MPR and oblique thin-MIP real-time visualization. Volume rendered images are occasionally useful for demonstrating structural relationships and unusual anatomic variants; however they are usually superfluous in routine image interpretation. Careful inspection of all coronary artery segments, cardiac, vascular, and noncardiovascular structures is undertaken in multiple planes, typically utilizing both oblique MPR and thin-MIP images. When analyzing CCTA images, it is important to select the image demonstrating the least apparent motion in a given phase series for a given coronary segment. It is crucial to understand the complexities of image acquisition to be able to navigate and manipulate the vast dataset typical of cardiac CTA. The finer details of CCTA interpretation are beyond the scope of this book.

1.4.3   Dose

Computing effective dose (E, mSv) in cardiac CT is a complex topic, which will be briefly summarized. The radiation output from a specific CT scanner may be measured utilizing a phantom (typically 32 cm for chest) and constitutes a weighted average of peripheral and central phantom multiple slice average doses over a z-axis collimation of 100 mm (CTDI volume). The CTDI is typically normalized for a 120 kv and 100 mAs scan. In order to estimate the entire dose for a complete CT exam the dose-length product (DLP) is used. The DLP takes into account the entire z-axis of the exam as well as all scans within the exam. DLP is accurate in both helical (any pitch) and sequential scans. DLP and CTDI do not specify patient dose, as they do not take into account patient size, gender, age, unique anatomy, and the specific body part scanned. DLP is simply a way of measuring radiation output for a given protocol, and thus a way to compare protocols to one another.

Patient dose depends both on innate technical parameters of the CT machine, the selected scan parameters, and specific patient characteristics. The effective dose is measured in milli-Sieverts (mSv), and takes into account both the absorbed dose (mGy) and the weighted sensitivities of tissues receiving the radiation. Effective dose (E) is linearly and directly proportional to both tube current (mAs) and z-axis length of the patient exposed. There is no simple relationship between patient dose and kVp, but a general rule of thumb is that reducing from 120 to 100 kVp (while keeping all else constant) yields a 50 % decrease in effective dose. To estimate patient dose, Monte Carlo methods are used to accurately measure the dose to single organ based on a given scanner's innate characteristic, the technique used (kV, mAs, etc.), and protocol performed (z-axis collimation, number of scans, etc.).

The effective dose is expressed as the sum of all organ doses, each weighted based on their radiation sensitivity as detailed by the ICRP 103 in 2007. This yields a constant with the units (mSv/mGy × cm²), or shorthand (E/DLP).

This constant is then multiplied by the DLP to yield the effective dose (E) in milli-sieverts. Although controversial and constantly in flux, the current conversion factor for a full chest CT is 0.014 mSv/mGy×cm². The current conversion factor for cardiac CT is considerably higher as described by Huda et al. [4].

The linear-no-threshold model is commonly accepted as the most accurate predictive model for the nondeterministic (stochastic) effects of ionizing radiation, specifically the risk of radiation induced cancer. It is partly based on calculating relative cancer risk in data points from atom bomb survivors who received 50 mSv or greater. However, the lack of study data points in the 1–50 mSv range lends some experts to believe the linear threshold model is not apropos for medical imaging.

Dose optimization strategies are beyond the scope of this chapter. However, in general the principle of ALARA (As Low As Reasonably Achievable) is always the goal in medical imaging. Common strategies include: (1) optimal patient preparation, (2) low kVp technique, (3) low mAs with automated exposure control or EKG-gated exposure, (4) tightly collimated z-axis prescription, (5) prospective triggering, (6) adaptive and model based iterative reconstruction algorithms, and (7) ensuring the appropriateness of the study.

References

1. Kalendar WA. Computed tomography. 3rd ed. Erlangen: Publicis Publishing; 2011.
2. Marmourian AC. CT imaging: practical physics, artifacts and pitfalls. New York: Oxford University Press; 2013.
3. Achenbach S, Arbab-Zadeh A, Cury RC, Poon M, Weigold WG. SCCT cardiovascular CT board prep. 2nd ed. Washington, DC: Society of Cardiovascular CT; 2011.
4. Huda W, Tipnis S, Sterzik A, Schoepf UJ. Computing effective dose in cardiac CT. Phys Med Biol. 2010; 55(13):3675–84.

Artifacts

Muzammil H. Musani and Eric J. Feldmann

2

When a reconstructed image does not faithfully reproduce a true representation of the actual object, an artifact is felt to have occurred. Common artifacts in CCTA include motion, slab/stacking, blooming, and photon starvation. A brief description of commonly encountered artifacts is provided in this chapter; for pictures please refer to the image section.

2.1 Motion Artifact

There are three causes of motion artifact in CCTA: (1) cardiac/coronary motion, (2) respiratory motion, and (3) patient complete body motion. Another computational cause of apparent "motion artifact" may occur during multisegment reconstruction when interbeat variation in the location of coronary artery segments leads to superimposition failure.

2.2 Coronary Motion Artifact

All images in CCTA demonstrate an element of coronary/cardiac motion artifact. Coronary/cardiac motion is complex, comprising multiple additive movements, which include squeezing [1]. The degree of apparent coronary motion on a CCTA image is a complex interplay between: (1) intrinsic patient-specific coronary movement, (2) the patient's heart rate, (3) timing of scanning, (4) hardware related capabilities

of the scanner, and (5) software/postprocessing capabilities of the image data. Since only the first variable is fixed, strategies to reduce cardiac motion focus on the latter four.

The patient's heart rate is lowered to preferably around 60 beats per minutes (bpm) for most single source scanners. Dual source and newer single source scanners may tolerate higher heart rates. Typically this is performed via the negative chronotropic effects of metoprolol via PO or IV routes.

Imaging during diastole, hopefully including diastasis (the time of maximal left ventricular dilatation and minimal coronary movement), is the ideal imaging time for CCTA. This is achieved typically by choosing a delay corresponding to a %R-R of around 70–80 % of the cardiac cycle, in patients with slow heart rates (around 60 bpm). In patients with higher heart rates, the phase of minimal coronary artery motion moves toward systole.

Technologically, improving the effective temporal resolution intrinsic to the hardware of the scanner is the second strategy. The minimal amount of data needed to create an image, typically 180° plus fan angle (in single source scanners) and the gantry rotation speed, dictates the temporal resolution of a scanner. Dual source scanners utilize two photon source-detector row elements set roughly 90° from each other in the x-y plane (same z-axis alignment), to allow only about 90° plus fan angle of rotation to acquire minimum amount of data needed for image reconstruction. Newer single source scanners can rotate at 200 msec/revolution.

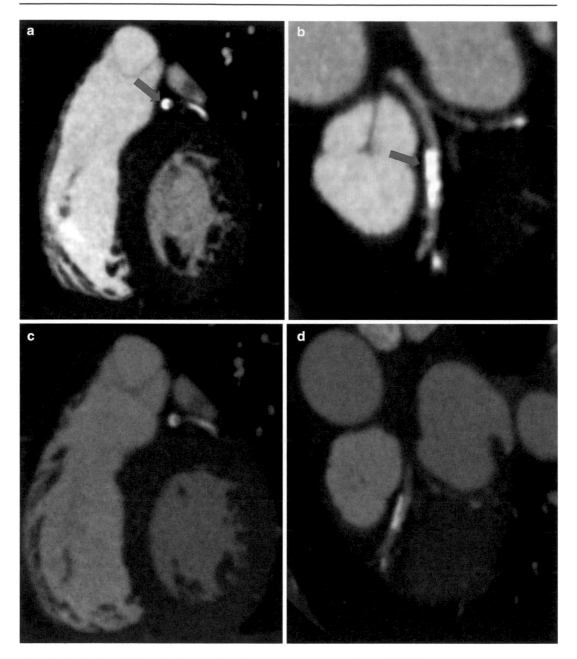

Fig. 2.1 (**a**, **b**) Non-MIP multiplanar reformations of "blooming artifact" in the LAD (*blue arrow*) from coronary artery calcium. This may be ameliorated using different scanning techniques as well as after image acquisition. (**c**, **d**) Manipulating window width and level/center in the DICOM viewer is a mandatory post-processing step in imaging interpretation. As window width increases the more "gray" the image becomes. Increasing window width may help "see behind" densely calcified plaque

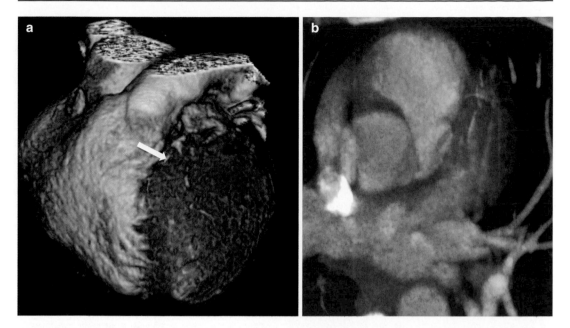

Fig. 2.2 (**a**, **b**) Patient's high heart rate, likely compounded by the patient's anatomy lending itself to a high velocity of coronary artery motion/translation, renders this phase uninterpretable. It is difficult to even see the LAD (*white arrow*) on the volume rendered image and axial maximum intensity projection image

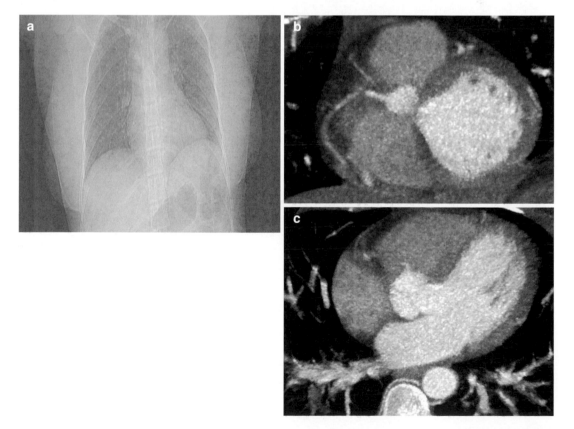

Fig. 2.3 Using low kVp can lead to increased noise (decreased signal-to-noise ratio (SNR)) in a patient with normal BMI. (**a**) Scout image gives an idea of chest wall width. (**b**, **c**) Coronary and axial maximum intensity projection images demonstrate a very grainy image limiting accurate assessment of patient's coronary artery stenosis

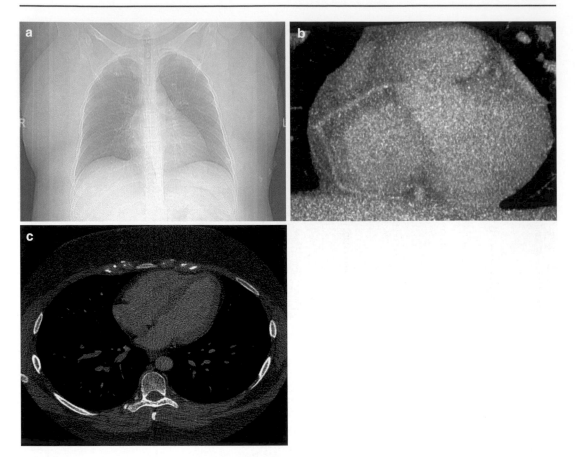

Fig. 2.4 (**a–c**) Using low kVp in obese patient may lead to a nondiagnostic study due to poor Signal to Noise Ratio (SNR). Compare images to Fig. 2.3. It is important to adjust parameters such as kVp and mAs prior to scanning obese patients

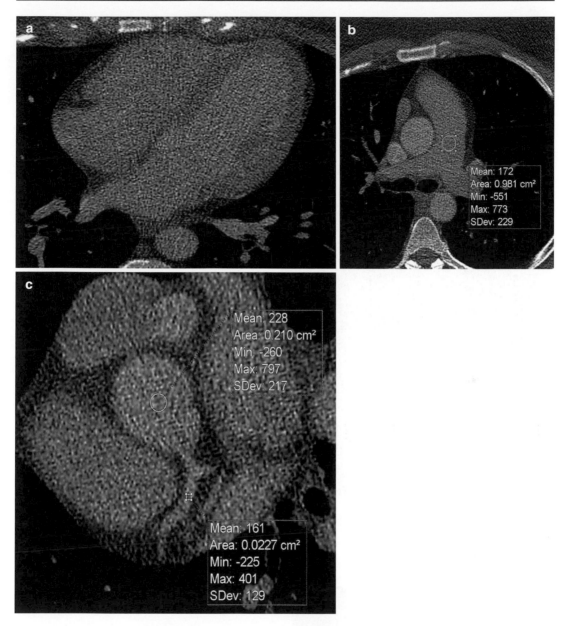

Fig. 2.5 (**a–c**) Multiplanar reformat images demonstrate poor quality due to poor contrast enhancement. Improper scanning parameters led to late scan initiation leading to suboptimal contrast enhancement of main pulmonary artery and coronary arteries. Also note poor signal-to-noise ratio

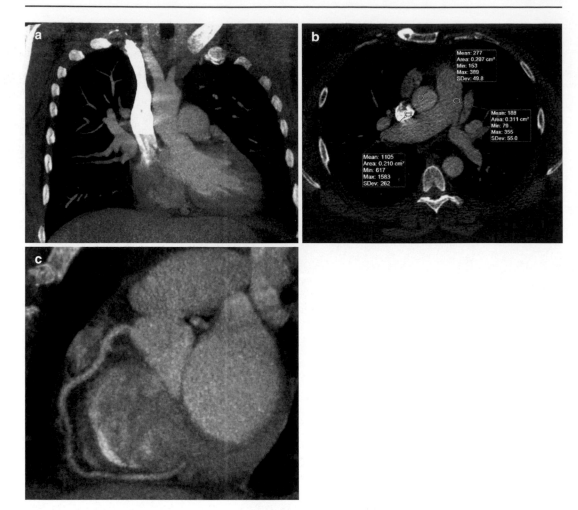

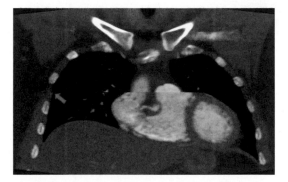

Fig. 2.6 (**a–c**) Multiplanar reformat images demonstrate suboptimal contrast enhancement of main pulmonary artery and coronary arteries contrast layering within the superior vena cava (SVC) consistent with early scan triggering. Typically, this would not be seen in a "late" scan

Fig. 2.7 Coronal maximum intensity projection image demonstrate improper stitching (*arrow*) in a 320-detector row scanner. It is similar to slab artifact in a 64 detector row scanner

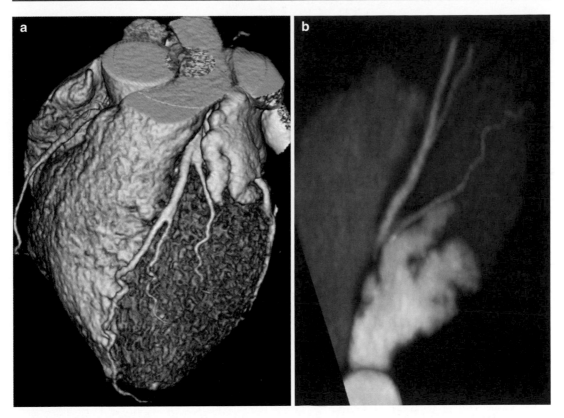

Fig. 2.8 (**a**, **b**) 3D volume rendered and maximum intensity projection images demonstrate distal tapering of the coronary vasculature. Patient took phosphodiesterase inhibitors prior to scanning and could not receive sublingual nitroglyc-erine. Poor vasodilation may lead to nondiagnostic image quality, particularly in patients with abundant calcified atheromata

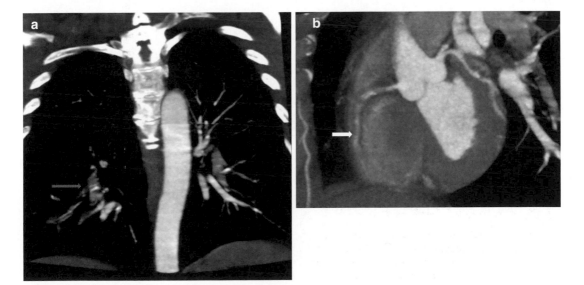

Fig. 2.9 (**a**, **b**) Coronal maximum intensity projection image demonstrates extensive motion of the pulmonary vasculature (*blue arrow*) and right coronary artery (*white arrow*), which was caused by patient respiratory motion. Respiratory motion may be confirmed by evaluating the lung bases and chest wall for misregistration. On the other hand, pulsation artifact should cause minimal motion of the central pulmonary arteries in an EKG gated study

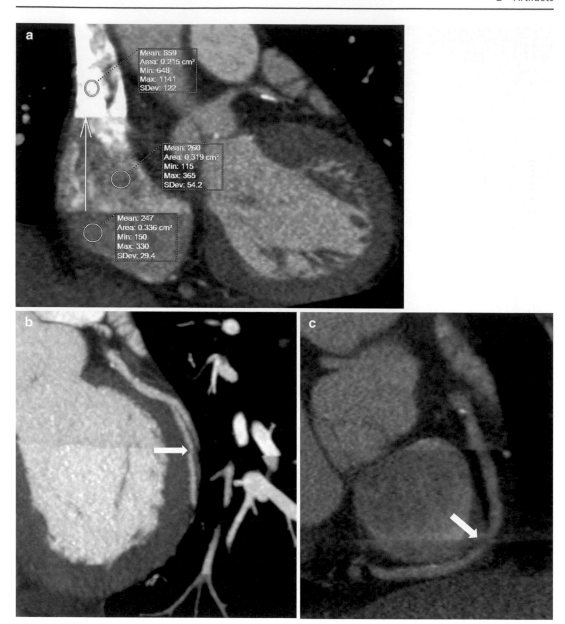

Fig. 2.10 (**a**) Coronal multiplanar reformation on a 64 detector row CT scanner utilizing step and shoot technique with prospective triggering demonstrates typical "slab artifact" or "misregistration artifact." This occurs due to slight differences in interbeat cardiac anatomy locations (i.e., the coronary artery does not wind up in the same location each beat). R-R interval variability also contributes to this artifact. (**b**, **c**) If a coronary artery is affected by slab artifact it can create a false impression of obstructive coronary artery disease (*white arrow*)

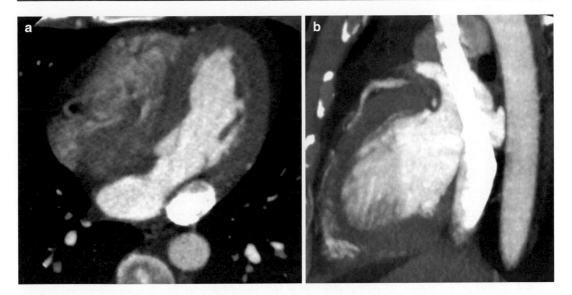

Fig. 2.11 (**a**, **b**) Axial and sagittal multiplanar reformat images demonstrate a persistent left-sided superior vena cava. Due to its close proximity to the descending aorta, scanning may be triggered early. If the bolus tracking method is used with an ROI in the adjacent descending thoracic aorta, "streak artifact" from the adjacent dramatically enhancing SVC may result in premature or late scan triggering

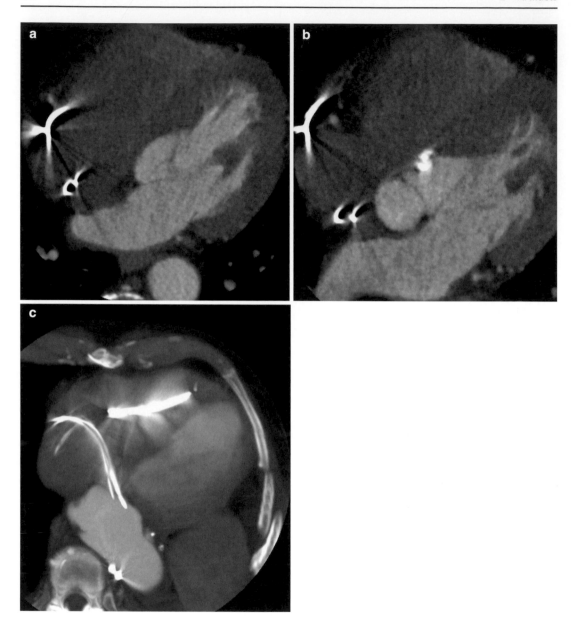

Fig. 2.12 (**a–b**) Demonstrates a pacing wire resulting in "streak artifact". (**c**) Demonstrates prominent streak artifact from an AICD shock coil in the right ventricle. "When an object attenuates nearly all photons, not only does it demonstrate an extremely high HU number, but it often results in the inability to accurately back project data along rays involved with the object. This results in "streaks" of low and high attenuation emanating from the structure along the rays affected"

References

1. Mao S, Lu B, Oudiz RJ, Bakhsheshi H, Liu SC, Budoff MJ. Coronary artery motion in electron beam tomography. J Comput Assist Tomogr. 2000; 24:253–8.

2. Liang Z, Karl WC, Do S, Brady T, Pien H. Analysis and mitigation of calcium artifacts in cardiac multidetector CT. IEEE Paris, France Conference International Symposium on Biomedical Imaging: from Nano to Macro, vol. 1–4; 2008. p. 1477–80.

3. Kruk M, Noll D, Achenbach S, Mintz G, et al. Impact of coronary artery calcium characteristics on accuracy of CT angiography. J Am Coll Cardiol Img. 2014;7(1):49–58.

4. Do S, Karl WC, Lian Z, Kalra M, Brady TJ, Pien HH. A decomposition-based CT reconstruction formulation for reducing blooming artifacts. Phys Med Biol. 2011;56(22):7109–25.

Cardiac CT in Adult Congenital Heart Disease

3

Muzammil H. Musani, Desiree M. Younes, and Eric J. Feldmann

3.1 Introduction

Cross-sectional cardiac imaging is increasingly being used to characterize congenital heart defects (CHD) and their associated extracardiac abnormalities. Both cardiac CT (CCT) and cardiac magnetic resonance imaging (CMR) are helpful in the diagnosis and monitoring of medically managed or surgically corrected CHD in adults. Additionally, clinically silent defects in young or middle-aged adults are often incidentally found with cross-sectional imaging done for unrelated purposes. Unlike CMR, CCT provides only morphological data. However, due to the relative availability, heightened spatial resolution, and short acquisition time of CCT, it is an important tool in the evaluation of CHD [1–5].

3.2 Normal Cardiac Anatomy

Describing complex congenital defects has been simplified by the development of a "sequential segmental" approach to cardiac imaging [1, 2, 6–8]. This approach utilizes morphological criteria, rather than spatial orientation, to describe CHD.

Cardiac situs is first determined; this is defined by the relative relation of the atria. The left and right atria are differentiated from each other by their appendages: the left atrial (LA) appendage has a narrow opening and finger-like projections, while the right atrial (RA) appendage has a broader base and is triangular shaped. The RA also has a crista and pectinate muscles [9].

Subsequently, each of the three cardiac segments (atria, ventricle, and great arteries) is located. The morphological right ventricle (RV) is triangular; it contains a moderator band and coarse muscular trabeculations along the interventricular septum. The RV also has a muscular infundibulum separating the atrioventricular valve from its semilunar valve. The left ventricle (LV) is elliptical, has fine trabeculations, and is with fibrous continuity between the atrioventircular (AV) and semilunar valves. The tricuspid valve consists of three leaflets (septal anterior, superior, and inferior), which are supported by papillary muscles that arise from the trabeculations of the RV. The mitral valve has two leaflets, each supported by a papillary muscle group. The great arteries are defined by their branches, and the great veins are defined by the organs that they drain.

The next step in the sequential segmental approach in describing cardiac structure is to determine venoatrial, atrioventricular (AV), and ventriculoarterial (VA) connections. Normally, the RA is connected to the RV through the tricuspid valve and the LA to the LV through the mitral valve. This is termed concordance. Abnormal AV connections include discordant connections, atresia of the AV valve, and double inlet ventricle (defined as over 50 % of each AV valve overlying a single, dominant ventricle) [2, 9, 10]. Abnormal VA connections include discordance, atresia,

M.H. Musani et al., *Clinical Pearls in Diagnostic Cardiac Computed Tomographic Angiography*,
DOI 10.1007/978-3-319-08168-7_3, © Springer International Publishing Switzerland 2015

double outlet ventricle, and the presence of a common arterial trunk (truncus arteriosus).

Associated cardiac anomalies should subsequently be identified. These include intracardiac anomalies, such as atrial and ventricular septal defects, as well as extracardiac anomalies, such as coarctation of the aorta, patent ductus arteriosus, and anomalous coronary arteries. The cardiac position within the chest and orientation of the apex should also be determined.

3.3   CHD in the Adult

Many types of CHD of simple to moderate complexity may not present until the second or third decade in life. In fact, at least 10 % of adults with CHD are not diagnosed until adulthood [11]. The incidental discovery of CHD on cross-sectional imaging done for noncardiac purposes is not uncommon [3]. Additionally, due to advances in pediatric cardiac care, 85 % of babies born with CHD are expected to reach adulthood [12]. Many of these patients do not establish cardiac follow-up when transitioning to adult care and may eventually present to regional cardiac centers [13]. Knowledge of the anatomy of CHD on cross-sectional imaging is important in the management of these patients.

3.4   Specific Congenital Heart Defects in the Adult

3.4.1   Atrial Septal Abnormalities

Atrial septal defects (ASD) are the most common congenital defect found in adults; they make up about 30 % of all lesions [14, 15]. The size of the shunt through the ASD increases with age, and by the age of 40, more than half of affected patients develop shortness of breath, fatigability, atrial arrhythmias, or, rarely, pulmonary hypertension [16–18].

Ostium secundum defects are the most common type of ASD, accounting for 75 % of defects. They are the result of a malformation of the fossa ovalis and are located centrally in the interatrial septum (IAS). Ostium primum defects, which account for 15 % of ASDs, occur at the site of the endocardial cushions in the lower part of the IAS. These defects are often associated with mitral and tricuspid regurgitation or ventricular septal defects. Sinus venosus defects make up 10 % of ASDs and result from the failure of the sinus venosus to incorporate into the right atrium. These defects occur at the junction of the superior or inferior vena cavae to the right atrium; the superior type is commonly associated with partially anomalous pulmonary venous return [2, 3, 16, 19, 20].

A patent foramen ovale (PFO) occurs when the septum primum and septum secundum, which normally fuse shortly after birth, remains patent [14]. This occurs in 20–34 % of people [21]. This defect is usually asymptomatic, although it can be associated with a range of illnesses such as migraines and sleep apnea. The most common presenting symptoms are related to paroxysmal emboli (stroke). An associated atrial septal aneurysm, defined as a redundancy in the IAS that results in a 10 mm protrusion of the septum beyond its plane [22], should be noted on cardiac imaging. The presence of an IAS aneurysm increases the risk of stroke and may affect the stability of percutaneous closure devices [16, 23].

Rarely, a defect in the roof of the coronary sinus may occur that leads to an abnormal communication between the LA and the coronary sinus. This results in intra-atrial left to right shunting similar to that seen with an ASD despite an intact IAS. An unroofed coronary sinus may be associated with a persistent left superior vena cava [20, 24].

Echocardiography is the imaging modality of choice in diagnosing ASDs as small defects may be missed on nongated cardiac CT [1]. However, cardiac CT can aid in assessing the size and location of a secundum ASD and its rims; this information is needed to determine the possibility of percutaneous, rather than surgical, closure [25, 26]. Sinus venosus ASDs, which are usually high in the IAS, may be missed on echocardiography and, along with anomalous pulmonary venous return, may require cross-sectional imaging for diagnosis.

Other atrial abnormalities, such as left atrial diverticulium and left atrial accessory appendages, are being diagnosed more often with the increased use of cardiac CT and likely represent normal variants [27–29]. LA diverticula have been reported in up to 36 % of patients undergoing cardiac CT; [29] 4.4 % of diverticula were noted on the IAS. Cardiac CT can also aid in the diagnosis of other benign structural heart defects. For example, lipomatous hypertrophy of the interatrial septum can be seen in up to 8 % of patients undergoing echocardiography and can lead to unnecessary invasive procedures [30–32]. On cardiac CT, this lesion appears as a mass of fat along the IAS that spares the fossa ovalis. The diagnosis of this lesion can be made with noninvasive cardiac imaging, rather than with invasive procedures [33].

3.4.2   Ventricular Septal Defects

Ventricular septal defect (VSD) is the most common cardiac congenital abnormality in children. With a prevalance of 0.08 %, it is the second most common cardiac congenital abnormality in adults (following ASD) [15]. Most VSDs close spontaneously by age 10; repair during childhood is considered only if associated with congestive heart failure (CHF) or pulmonary hypertension [19, 20]. VSDs that present in adulthood are usually small and without symptoms. If large enough, however, they can result in CHF or pulmonary hypertension [16].

The interventricular septum (IVS) is composed of an inlet, trabecular, and outlet components which surround a small, membranous septum at the base of the heart [9, 34]. Membranous VSDs make up 70 % of all VSDs [16]. These VSDs are bordered at least in part by fibrous continuity of an AV or arterial valve but may extend into the muscular septum. Muscular VSDs make up 20 % of all defects and are located in the trabecular septum, which extends from the membranous septum to the apex. The inlet portion of the IVS is located between the AV valves and their chordal attachments. Inlet

VSDs are associated with other defects of the AV canal. Defects in the infundibular septum, which separates the right and left ventricular outflow tracts and is bordered superiorly by the semilunar valves, may result from malalignment and is more frequently seen with other CHDs such as tetralogy of Fallot.

Cross-sectional imaging serves a complementary role to echocardiography in assessing VSDs. Cardiac CT can be used to assess less common VSDs, such as inlet or apical VSDs, as well as to evaluate the pulmonary vasculature [16, 35].

3.4.3   Bicuspid Aortic Valve

Bicuspid aortic valve (BAV) is seen in 0.5–2 % of the population, more commonly in men [3, 9]. BAV results from abnormal development of the aortic valve commissures and fusion of the coronary cusps; 70–80 % of cases involve the right and left cusps. Symptoms are rare until the fourth or fifth decade of life, when the progressive valve calcification that results from turbulent blood flow leads to significant aortic stenosis (AS) or aortic insufficiency (AI) [3, 20].

CCT is useful in patients with BAV. Accurate measurements of the ascending aorta, which is frequently dilated in those with significant AS or AI, are needed prior to aortic valve replacement as concomitant aortic root replacement may need to be considered. Additionally, it allows for noninvasive assessment of coronary artery disease prior to open heart surgery. CCT can also asses for coarctation of the aorta, which is commonly associated with BAV.

3.4.4   Quadricuspid Aortic Valve

Quandricuspid aortic valve is rare congenital AV abnormality that leads to significant valvular disease in adulthood. It is found in up to 0.04 % of the general population but in 1 % of those undergoing surgery for "pure" AI [36, 37]. Fibrous thickening of the leaflets leads to incomplete coaptation and AI. Surgery is often required by the fifth or sixth decade of life [38].

3.4.5   Pulmonary Valve Abnormalities

Pulmonary stenosis makes up 10–12 % of cases of adult CHD. Valvular stenosis results from varying degrees of commissural fusion and is responsible for 90 % of cases [9, 19]. Adults with mild RV outflow tract obstruction often have no symptoms, but 20 % of those with moderate obstruction progress and develop evidence of right sided volume overload [39]. Intervention is indicated when peak pressure gradient surpasses 60 mmHg or when symptoms are present. Percutaneous balloon valvuloplasty is the treatment of choice [20].

Quadricuspid pulmonary valves are five times more common than quadricuspid aortic valves and develop from a partitioning of one of the three embryologic valve cushions during early valvulogenesis [40, 41]. When isolated, quadricuspid pulmonic valves are clinically silent and are diagnosed incidentally.

3.4.6   Ebstein's Anomaly

Ebstein's anomaly (EA) is rare, occurring in 1 out of 200,000 live births [42]. Failure of the septal and posterior leaflets of the tricuspid valve to delaminate from the underlying myocardium during fetal development results in apical displacement of the tricuspid annulus and "atrialization" of the right ventricle. This results in varying degrees of tricuspid regurgitation, and right atrial enlargement results [9]. An ASD is present in 50–94 % of patients due to atrial enlargement and gaping of a PFO [9, 42, 43].

Patients with only moderate tricuspid disease may not develop symptoms until early adulthood. These patients may develop arrhythmias, exercise intolerance, cyanosis, or right-sided heart failure. They are also at risk for paradoxical embolization through existing ASDs and brain abscesses [42, 44]. The diagnosis is usually made on echocardiography. Surgical repair of the tricuspid valve is indicated in patients that develop cyanosis, right-sided heart failure, decrease in functional capacity, and recurrent emboli. Relative indications for repair include asymptomatic cardiomegaly and recurrent atrial arrhythmias.

3.4.7   Patent Ductus Arteriosus

The ductus arteriosus is an arterial structure that connects the proximal left pulmonary artery to the descending aorta, just distal to the left subclavian artery. During fetal development, it serves to reroute deoxygenated blood from the RV to the aorta for oxygenation by the placenta. Normally, oxygen causes the duct to vasoconstriction and functionally close within 72 h of birth. In about 1 in 500 children, the duct fails to close; this is termed patent ductus arteriosus (PDA) [9, 14, 16, 45].

Small to moderate PDAs may remain silent or may present in adulthood as systemic arterial resistance rises and increases shunting to the pulmonary vasculature. Presenting features include pulmonary vascular congestion, atrial arrhythmias from LA enlargement, and endarteritis. The development of Eisenmenger's syndrome may result in shunting of pulmonary arterial blood into the aorta distal to the left subclavian artery. This leads to cyanosis or clubbing of the lower extremities only, termed "differential cyanosis" [14, 45]. Clinical symptoms, volume overload, and endarteritis are indications for PDA closure.

Echocardiography can establish the diagnosis and assess for elevated pulmonary pressures and cardiac chamber enlargement. CCT is used to noninvasively characterize the size, morphology, and calcifications of the ductus. This information is needed for selecting the modality of closure (open versus transcatheter) and the size of the closure device [46].

3.4.8   Coarctation of the Aorta

Coarctation of the aorta is a narrowing of the aorta, usually between the left subclavian artery and the ductus arteriosus, due to a localized shelf in the aortic well or tubular hypoplasia of the aorta. Collateral vessels are often present, and some patients do not present until early adulthood. Hypertension in the upper extremities is common.

Long-term complications are due to severe hypertension and include cerebral aneurysms and hemorrhage, hypertensive encephalopathy, aortic rupture, LV failure, and endocarditis [1, 2, 9].

Cross-sectional imaging establishes the diagnosis, degree and morphology of stenosis, and presence of collateral vessels [47, 48]. Repair is indicated when the gradient across the lesion is under 20 mmHg or when collateral vessels are present and often can be done with percutaneous stenting [20]. Postoperative monitoring with cross-sectional imaging is necessary to screen for complications such as restenosis and aneurysm formation [3, 9]. Metallic clips and stents cause streak artifact on MR; CT is often more useful in the postoperative patient.

3.4.9 Partial Anomalous Pulmonary Venous Return

Partial anomalous pulmonary venous return (PAPVR) is the drainage of one or more of the pulmonary veins directly or indirectly into the right atrium, seen in 0.3 % of adults [16]. In 79 % of cases presenting in adults, the left upper lobe of the lung drains to a left vertical vein, which drains into a dilated left brachiocephalic vein [49]. Only 17 % of adult cases involved drainage of the right upper lobe into the superior vena cava; patients with this anatomy, which is associated with sinus venosus ASD, may present at an earlier age. The pulmonary veins may also drain into the azygos vein or the coronary sinus. Pulmonary drainage into the inferior vena cava is termed scimitar syndrome and is associated with hypoplasia and abnormal arterial collateral supply of the right lung as well as dextrocardia [2, 9, 16].

Patients with PAPVR do not develop symptoms unless over 50 % of pulmonary return is anomalous or unless an ASD is present. View of the pulmonary veins may be limited on echocardiography; cardiac CT is helpful in establishing the diagnosis [50]. Associated abnormalities, such as enlargement of the right heart and pulmonary artery, can also be seen on CT [49]. Surgical intervention should be considered in cases of right ventricular volume overload [9].

3.4.10 Anomalous Systemic Venous Return

Persistence of the left superior vena cava (SVC), which results from failure of the left anterior cardinal vein to regress during fetal development, is seen in under 0.5 % of the general population and in 4 % of those with CHD [51]. When isolated, the left SVC usually drains into the coronary sinus. A right SVC is frequently present, and the two cavae may be connected by an anterior bridging vein [2]. When associated with CHD, it may drain into the LA [52]. Although this condition is not normally associated with symptoms, it may result in difficulties with placement of intravenous lines or intracardiac devices.

Other systemic venous anomalies in the thorax include abnormal drainage or dilation of the right SVC, abnormal course of the left brachiocephalic vein, and abnormal drainage of the inferior vena cava. These anomalies are rare and, when isolated, clinically silent [51].

3.4.11 Aortopulmonary Collaterals

Aortopulmonary collaterals (APCs) are remnants of embryonic ventral splanchnic arteries arising from the systemic arteries that provide blood to the pulmonary circulation [53, 54]. They are seen most commonly with cyanotic lesions, such as tetralogy of Fallot with pulmonary atresia and single ventricle heart disease, and the majority is found during infancy [55]. They can be newly diagnosed in adults and are associated with right lung hypoplasia. Their presence and the territory that they supply are important factors when considering shunt placement and other cardiac surgeries [2, 53].

3.4.12 Tetralogy of Fallot Repair

Tetralogy of Fallot (ToF) is the most common cyanotic CHD seen in adults. Malalignment of the septal components of the fetal heart leads to an overlying aorta, RV outflow tract (RVOT) obstruction, VSD, and RV hypertrophy. The degree of left-to-right shunting is determined by the severity of the RVOT obstruction. Most patients present shortly after birth, and without surgical correction, there is a near 90 % mortality by age 20 [9, 56, 57].

In the past, surgical repair was accomplished by creating conduits between the systemic and pulmonary artery (PA). Anastomosis can be created between the ascending aorta and right PA (Waterston operation), descending aorta to left PA (Potts operation), or subclavian artery to main PA (Blalock–Taussig operation). Currently, complete ToF repair is performed and consists of closure of the VSD and relieve of RVOT obstruction [56].

With surgery, the majority of patients live well into adulthood [58]. Postoperative complications include residual VSD or RVOT obstruction, pulmonary insufficiency that may lead to RV failure, or PA stenosis. CCT is useful for postoperative assessment of the PA and RV. CCT can also be used to evaluate cardiac defects associated with ToF, seen in 68 % of patients, such as right aortic arch and anomalous coronary arteries [1, 43, 59].

3.4.13 Congenital Absence of Pericardium

Congenital absence of pericardium is extremely rare, with only cases reported in the literature. The defect may be partial or complete, and it may be associated with other cardiac defects such as ASD or bicuspid aortic valve. Symptoms, if present, are most often sharp, paroxysmal chest pains. Life-threatening complications include torsion of the great vessels and herniation of portions of the heart through the defect [9, 60, 61].

Imaging reveals leftward shifting of the apex, right ventricular enlargement, and the presence of lung tissue between the aorta and left PA. MR can directly visualize the pericardium and confirm the presence and extent of the defect [62, 63]. Surgical reconstruction of the pericardium is considered in symptomatic patients.

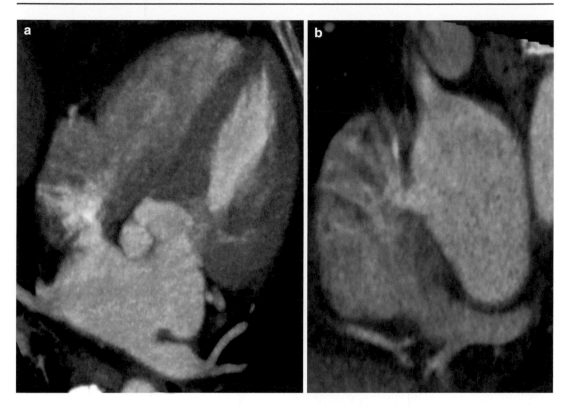

Fig. 3.1 (**a**) Axial near- four chamber maximum intensity projections at the level of the aortic root demonstrates left atrial contrast passing through a defect in the interatrial septum and into the right atrium. *These findings are consistent with an atrial septal defect and should be corroborated with other projections and phases. In general,* *admixture artifact must be excluded, although it is typically not this robust.* (**b**) Near short axis oblique multiplanar reformat at the level of the interatrial septum confirms left atrial contrast passing through a defect in the interatrial septum and into the right atrium. The location is most consistent with an ostium secundum defect

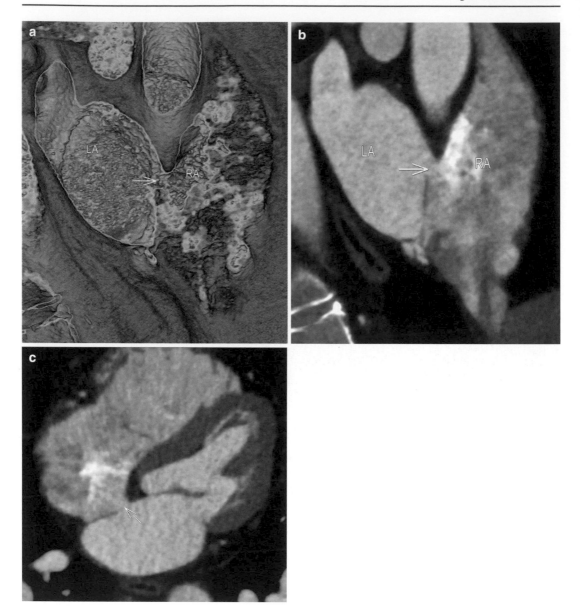

Fig. 3.2 (a) Near-short axis hollow volume rendered image at the level of the superior interatrial septum demonstrates a connection between with left atrium and right atrium, which is located far anteriorly (*white arrow*). (b) An oblique multiplanar reformat at the same level confirms this (*arrow*). *Notice that the right atrium demonstrates prominent admixture artifact, as is typical. No prominent left to right contrast jet is present in this case,* *due to differences in contrast timing when compared to the first case.* (c) Oblique multiplanar reformatted four chamber image at the superior aspect of the interatrial septum delineates the ostium primum defect (*arrow*). Note, how the contrast at the far left aspect of the right atrium is similar in attenuation to the left atrium, and is free of admixture artifact. *LA* left atrium, *RA* right atrium

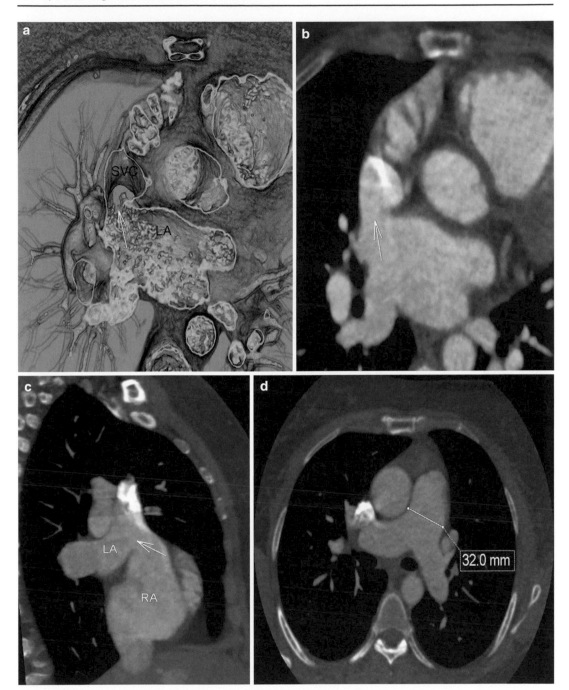

Fig. 3.3 (**a**) Near axial projection hollow volume rendered image at the level of the superior vena cava/left atrium. Image demonstrates a connection between the far superior left atrium and the base of the superior vena cava at its entry to the right atrium (*white arrow*) consistent with a sinus venosus type atrial septal defect (superior vena cava type). (**b**) Oblique multiplanar reformat in the same projection demonstrates fairly homogenous contrast between the superior vena cava and the left atrium (*arrow*), with slight high attenuation admixture artifact from the continued injection of intravenous contrast. (**c**) Near sagittal oblique multiplanar reformat at the level of the right atrium demonstrates the left atrium connected to the superior vena cava at its insertion to the right atrium (*white arrow*). (**d**) Axial multiplanar *reformat demonstrates an enlarged main pulmonary at 32 mm (normal up to 29 mm), which suggests pulmonary arterial hypertension in this patient with known left to right shunt physiology. SVC superior vena cava, LA left atrium, RA right atrium*

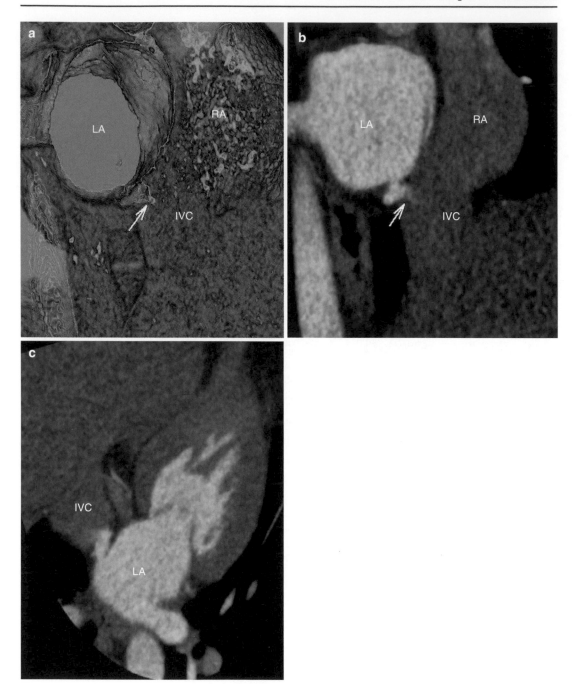

Fig. 3.4 (**a**) Oblique hollow volume rendered image and (**b**) Maximum Intensity Projection at the level of Inferior vena cava (*IVC*)/left atrium (*LA*) demonstrate a connection between inferomedial wall of the left atrium and the base of inferior vena cava (*IVC*) (*arrow*). (**c**) Maximum intensity projection image in an oblique near four chamber at the level of inferior atrial septum demonstrates a contrast jet traversing the posterior aspect of the interatrial septum and entering the far cranial aspect of the inferior vena cava- diagnostic of an sinus venosus ASD (inferior vena cava subtype)

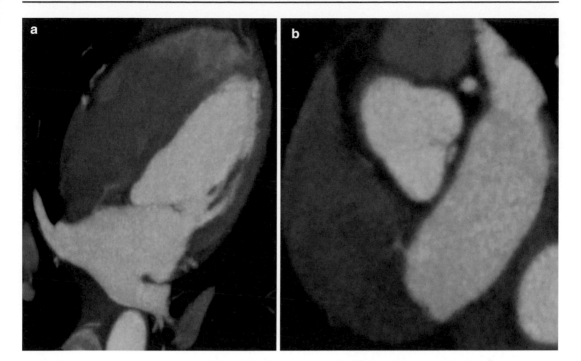

Fig. 3.5 (a) Near four-chamber maximum intensity projection at the left of the mid interatrial septum demonstrates a thin area of high attenuation contrast extending from the left atrium and passing through a small defect in the mid-interatrial septum, most consistent with a patent foramen ovale. *This finding is easily seen when there is a prominent difference in attenuation between the left atrium and right atrium, as is typically seen with modest contrast administration (40–70 ml) and excellent right atrial contrast nulling from a saline chaser.* (b) Near short axis multiplanar reformation at the level of the interatrial septum confirms a small defect in the mid-interatrial septum consistent with a patent foramen ovale

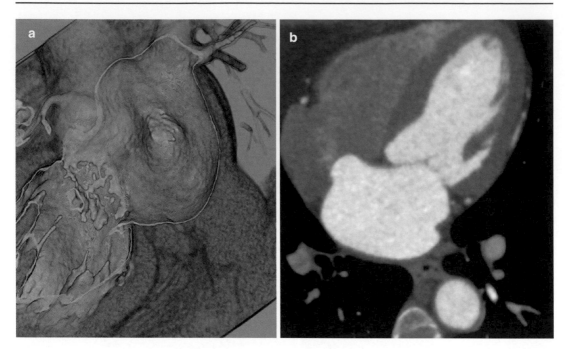

Fig. 3.6 (**a**) Volume rendered hollow image in a near two-chamber/long-axis projection of the left atrial lumen demonstrates a bulge of the interatrial septum away from the lumen- thus toward the right atrium. Findings are consistent with an atrial septal aneurysm. Typically these need to bulge 10 mm into the right atrium beyond the atrial septum, and are more accurately measured when there is continuous image acquisition throughout the cardiac cycle, as in echocardiography or MRI. (**b**) Oblique multiplanar reformation in a four chamber view demonstrates a prominent right-convex bulge of the interatrial septum, meeting criterion for an interatrial septal aneurysm, even on this static image in diastole. These are commonly associated with atrial septal defects, usually patent foramen ovale, which is suggested by the area of high attenuation contrast in the adjacent right atrium. This should be confirmed with other phases/projection and echocardiography

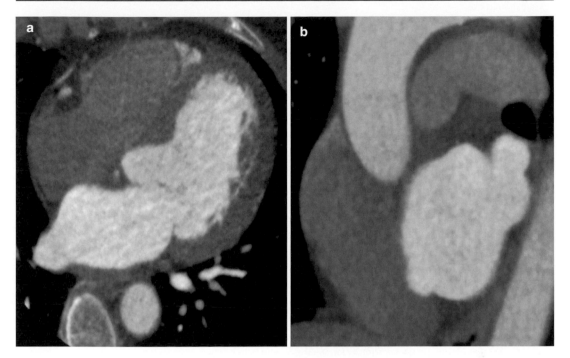

Fig. 3.7 (**a**) Oblique multiplanar reformation in a four chamber view demonstrates right-convex bulging of the interatrial septum suggesting an interatrial septal diverticulum, (**b**) a near short axis view confirms the right convex bulge in the mid portion of the atrial septum

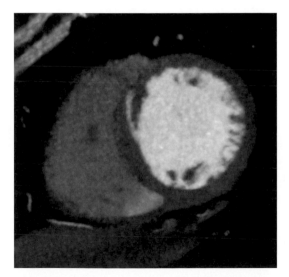

Fig. 3.8 A short axis maximum intensity projection at the level of the mid left ventricle demonstrates a deep trabeculation with the septum, which is continuous with the left ventricular lumen as demonstrated by robust contrast filling. A thin sliver of myocardium prevents contrast from filling the right ventricle, rendering the diagnosis of intramuscular ventricular septal defect unlikely. *These findings are most consistent with a diverticulum, however should be confirmed in multiple planes and phases*

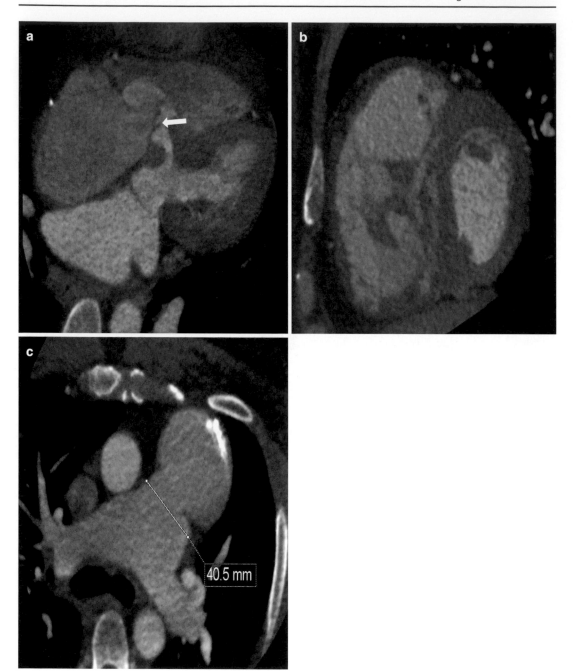

Fig. 3.9 (**a**) Near four-chamber maximum intensity projection just inferior to the membranous ventricular septum demonstrates a contrast filled defect in the peri-membranous interventricular septum. The vast majority of the defect is covered by a patch from prior surgical repair; however a thin sliver of contrast enters the right ventricle consistent with a persistent tiny communication between the left and right ventricles with left to right shunting (*white arrow*). (**b, c**) Oblique multiplanar reformations in short axis at the level of the mid left ventricle demonstrate as well as prominent right ventricular trabeculation and dilatation consistent with remodeling from chronic elevated right heart pressures. There is a D-shaped left ventricular cavity and dilatation of the main pulmonary artery (4.1 cm) suggesting elevated right heart pressures. These findings are the result of chronic remodeling and do not necessarily reflect the patient's current physiology

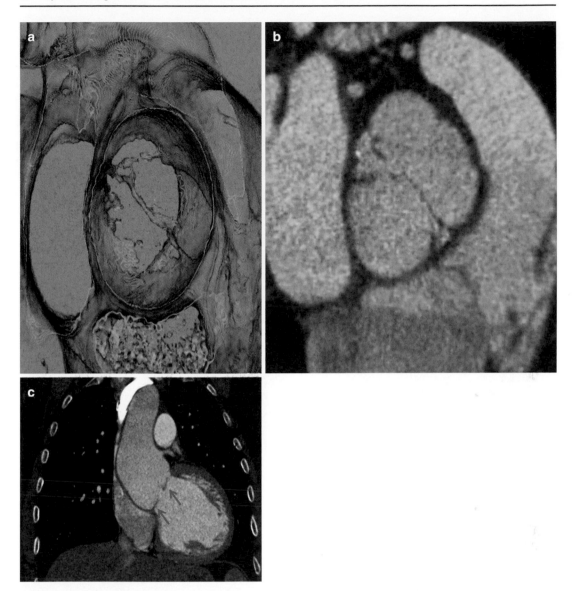

Fig. 3.10 (**a**, **b**) Volume rendered hollow and maximum intensity projection image of congenitally bicuspid aortic valve. (**c**) Oblique multiplanar reformat in a paracoronal LVOT plane demonstrates the bicuspid aortic valve with aneurysmal dilatation of the aortic root, effacement of the normal sinotubular junction offset and gradual tapering of the ascending aorta (*blue arrows*)

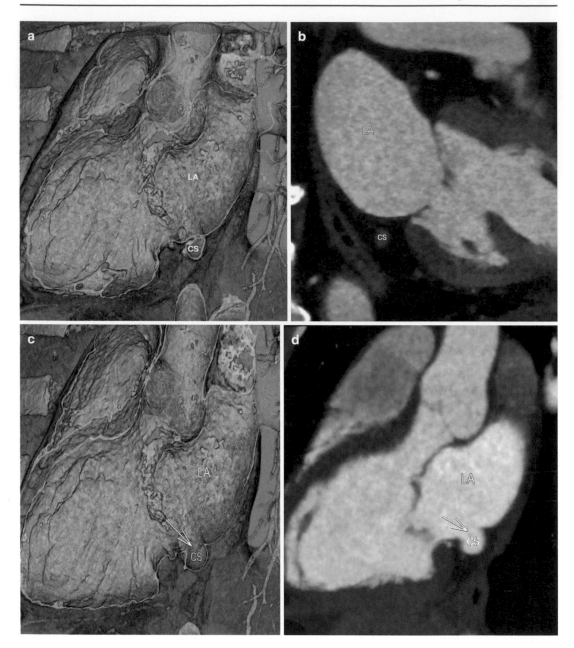

Fig. 3.11 (**a**) Volume rendered three chamber image demonstrates an intact roof of the coronary sinus (*CS*) with separation between it and the left atrium (*LA*). (**b**) Oblique multiplanar reformation in a two chamber long axis view demonstrates a normal area of fat interposed between the coronary sinus and the left atrium with normal poor contrast enhancement of the coronary sinus and robust left cardiac chamber enhancement. The coronary veins have yet to receive contrast from the myocardium, which account for the lack of coronary sinus enhancement. (**c**) Volume rendered three chamber image demonstrates a deficient roof of the coronary sinus (*arrow*) with resultant continuity between it and the left atrium. (**d**) Oblique multiplanar reformation in a three chamber view demonstrates connection between the coronary sinus and the left atrium (*arrow*) with resultant identical, homogeneous contrast enhancement of both chambers

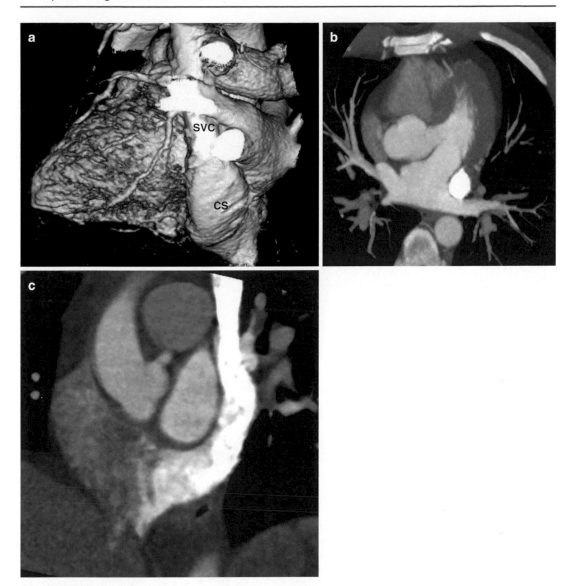

Fig. 3.12 (a) Volume rendered image in a near sagittal/ RAO projection demonstrates a vertical contrast filled vessel draining into a dilated coronary sinus (*CS*). These findings are diagnostic of a left-sided superior vena cava (*SVC*). (b) Maximum intensity projection in the axial plane at the level of the aortic root demonstrates an intravenous contrast filled vessel abutting the left border of the left atrium just anterior to the left inferior pulmonary vein. This is a typical location for a left sided superior vena cava. (c) Oblique multiplanar reformation in short axis at the level of the coronary sinus demonstrates a vertical contrast filled vessel draining into a dilated coronary sinus. These findings are diagnostic of a left-sided superior vena cava. The coronary sinus then mixes with unopacified blood in the right atrium from inferior vena cava return. This patient's intravenous contrast was injected via a left sided intravenous line

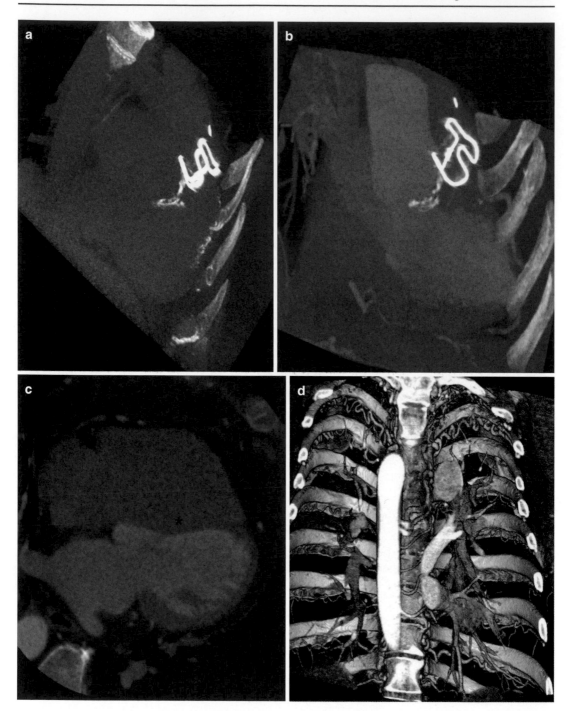

Fig. 3.13 (**a**) Oblique maximum intensity projection in a near RVOT plane demonstrates a bio-prosthetic valve in the pulmonary position, consistent with treatment of the Tetralogy of Fallot patient's pulmonic stenosis. (**b**) Oblique maximum intensity projection in a near LVOT plane demonstrates suture material in the area of the membranous ventricular septum consistent with ventriculoseptal defect repair in this patient with history of Tetralogy of Fallot. Re-demonstrated is the bio-prosthetic valve in the pulmonary position. (**c**) Oblique multiplanar reformat in a four chamber projection demonstrates dilated right heart chambers and a flattened interventricular septum (*) consistent with remodeling from elevated right side pressure. The ventricular septum is now intact. (**d**) Volume rendered coronary image of the entire thorax at the level of the descending aorta demonstrates dilated tortuous intercostal vessels/major aortopulmonary collateral arteries, which were the source of blood flow to the lungs in this patient with pulmonary artery atresia/stenosis

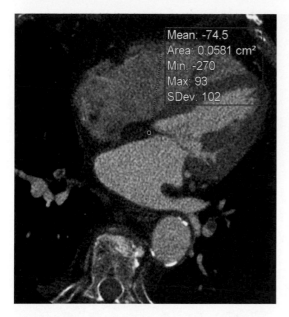

Mean: -74.5
Area: 0.0581 cm²
Min: -270
Max: 93
SDev: 102

Fig. 3.14 Oblique multiplanar reformation in a four chamber view demonstrates prominent tissue within the interatrial septum, with Hounsfield Unit attenuation consistent with simple fat. The typical criterion for lipomatous hypertrophy of the interatrial septum is: fat in the atrial septum at the level of the fossa ovalis measuring at least 2 cm in thickness

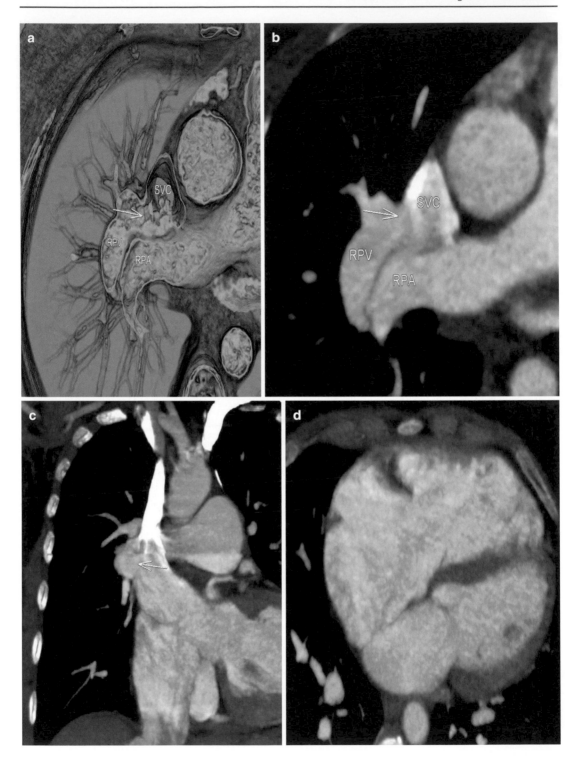

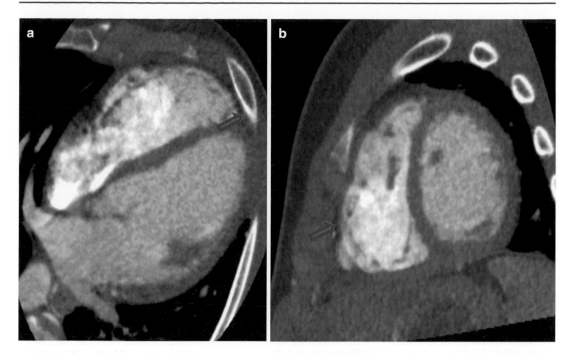

Fig. 3.16 (**a**, **b**) Oblique multiplanar reformation in a near four chamber and short axis view demonstrates epicardial fat abutting the anterior chest wall (*blue arrow*), and no clear evidence of the pericardium

Fig. 3.15 (**a**) Volume rendered hollow projection in the axial plane at the level of the superior vena cava (*SVC*) demonstrates anamolous connection of the right upper pulmonary vein (*RPV*) and the superior vena cava (*SVC*) (*white arrow*) diagnostic of partial anomalous pulmonary venous return, a left to right shunt. (**b**, **c**) Corresponding multiplanar reformat images in the axial plane and coronal plane demonstrates Anamolous connection of the right upper pulmonary vein and the superior vena cava (*white arrow*) diagnostic of partial anomalous pulmonary venous return, a left to right shunt. (**d**) Four chamber maximum intensity projection image demonstrates flattening of the interventricular septum and dilation of the right ventricle and atrium consistent with increased right sided pressures from left to right shunt. *RPA* right pulmonary artery

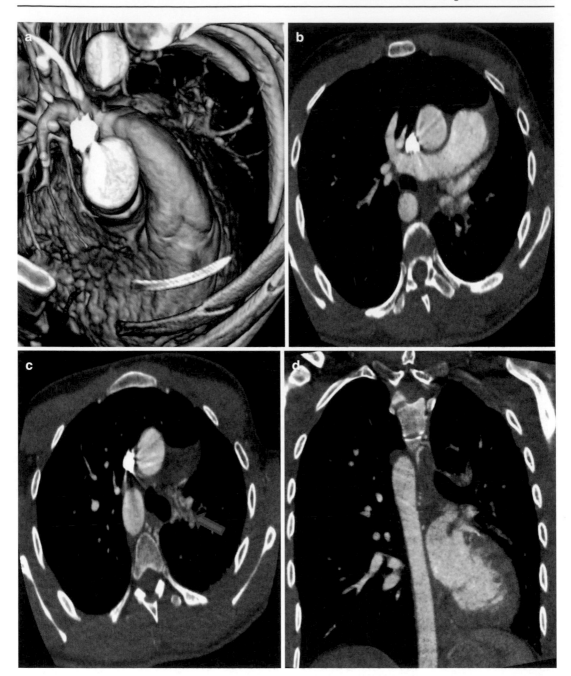

Fig. 3.17 (**a**) Caudally oriented near axial volume rendered image demonstrates absence of a normal left pulmonary artery. (**b**) Oblique multiplanar image in the near axial plane at the level of the main pulmonary artery demonstrates absence of the left pulmonary artery in the setting of a hypo plastic left lung and few small tortuous vessels adjacent to the left atrial appendage, consistent with major aortopulmonary collaterals. (**c**) Multiplanar image in the axial plane at the level of the aortic arch demonstrates numerous tortuous vessels adjacent to the left main stem bronchus and anterior to the vertebral body consistent with major aortopulmonary collaterals (*blue arrow*). (**d**) Multiplanar image in the coronal plane at the level of the descending aorta also demonstrates numerous tortuous vessels adjacent to the left mainstream bronchus and at the left aspect of the aorta consistent with major aortopulmonary collaterals. The left lung is hypoplastic

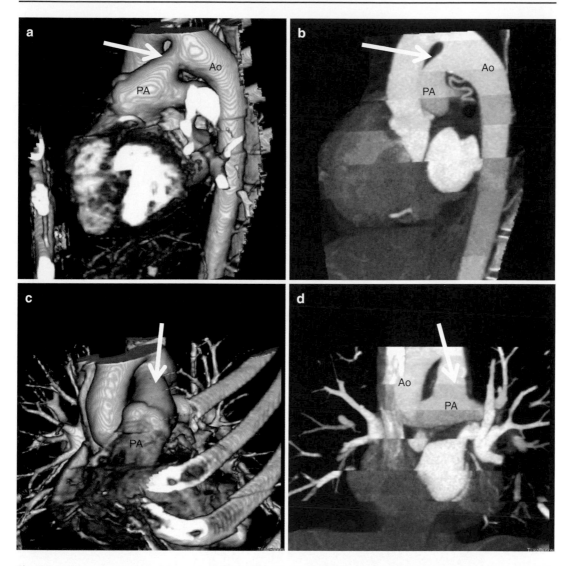

Fig. 3.18 3D volume rendered (**a**, **c**, **e**), oblique sagittal (**b**, **d**, **f**) reconstructions from two separate coronary CT angiograms demonstrating persistent postnatal patency of the ductus arteriosus (*white arrows*), which connects the main pulmonary artery (*PA*) and descending aorta (*Ao*). Cardiac MRI should be done to assess the severity of left to right shunt

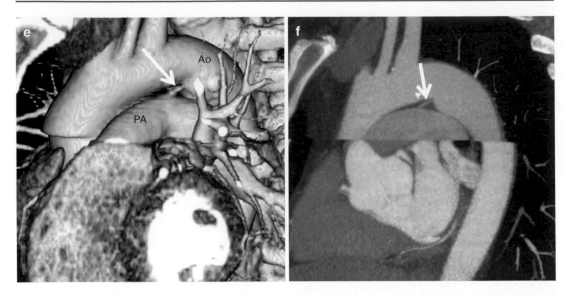

Fig. 3.18   (continued)

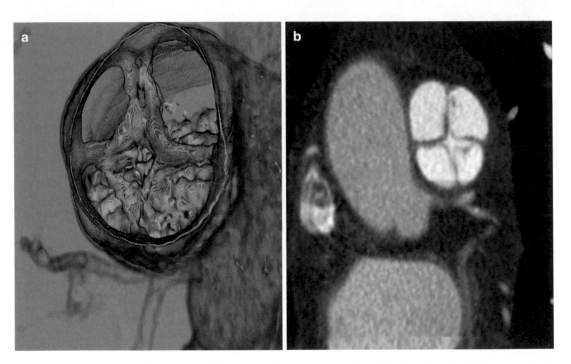

Fig. 3.19   (**a**, **b**) Volume rendered and multiplanar image demonstrate quadricuspid pulmonic valve. (**c**) Cross sectional multiplanar reformat image of a quadricuspid aortic valve

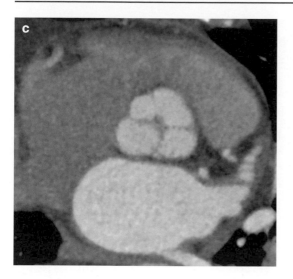

Fig. 3.19 (continued)

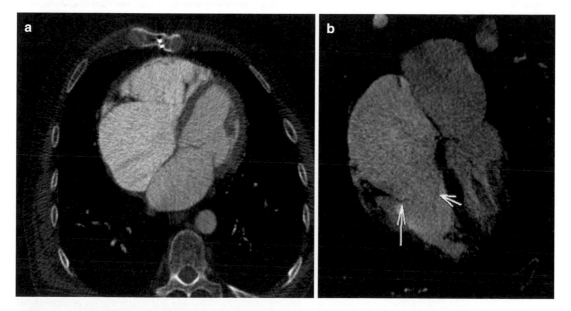

Fig. 3.20 (**a, b**) Multiplanar image in axial and four chamber view demonstrate septal displacement of tricuspid valve leaflets (*white arrow*), most consistent with Epstein's anomaly. To identify anomalous origin of coronary arteries the imager must get a good cross-sectional view of the aortic root. Should keep the slice thickness to a minimum of ≤2 mm

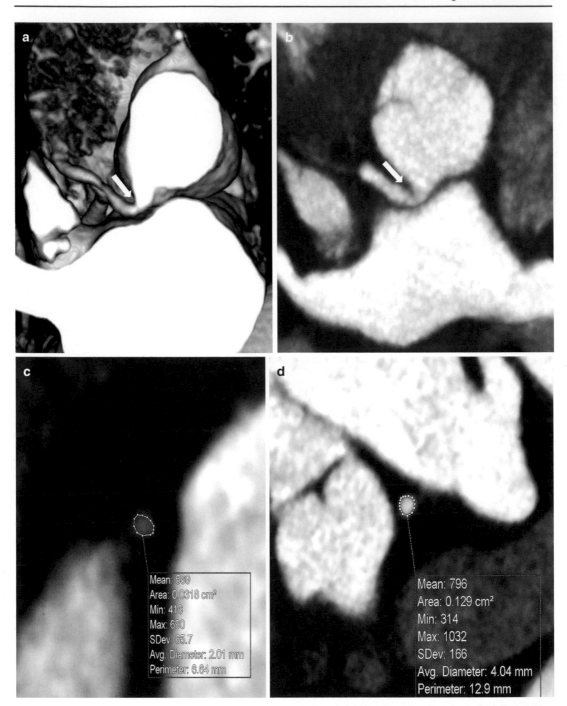

Fig. 3.21 (**a**) Volume rendered and multiplanar reformat (**b**) images of the aortic valve cranially demonstrates left main originating from the left coronary cusp, it has a sharp bend in the mid segment (*white arrow*). This bend reduces cross-sectional area of 50 % (**c**), when compared to cross-sectional area distal to the bend (**d**). Patient had presented to the ED for chest pain, CTA revealed no coronary artery disease. Patient had an inpatient stress test suggestive of reversible ischemia and went on for coronary artery bypass graft

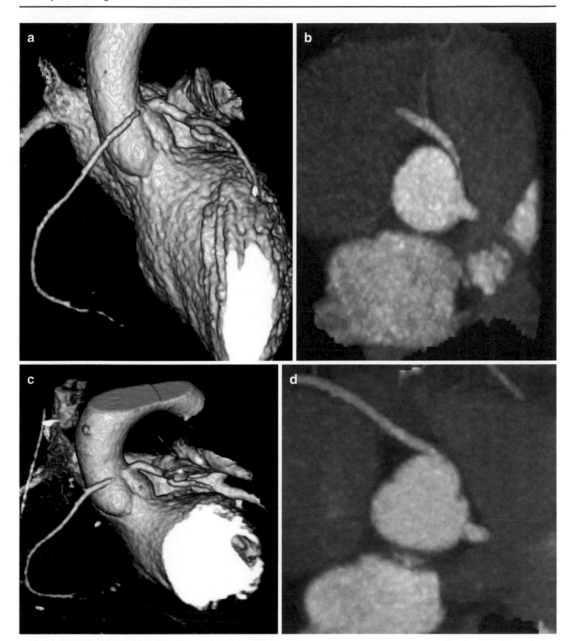

Fig. 3.22 (**a**) *Pre-Operative* Volume rendered caudal anterior oblique image of 15 year old male heart demonstrates an anomalous right coronary artery origin from the left Sinus of Valsalva with an aberrant retro pulmonic, pre aortic course. (**b**) Axial maximum intensity projection (MIP) image at the level of the Sinus of Valsalva demonstrates a possibly obstructive stenosis at the origin of the anomalous right coronary artery. *Patient underwent reimplantation of his RCA after having a positive stress* *echocardiogram.* (**c**) *Post-Operative* Volume rendered caudal anterior oblique image of the heart demonstrates the right coronary artery now emanating from the right Sinus of Valsalva in this patient status post reimplantation procedure. There is vague visualization of a rectangular patch at the sinotubular junction. (**d**) Axial maximum intensity projection (MIP) image at the level of the Sinus of Valsalva demonstrates normotopic origin of the right coronary artery from the right Sinus of Valsalva without stenosis

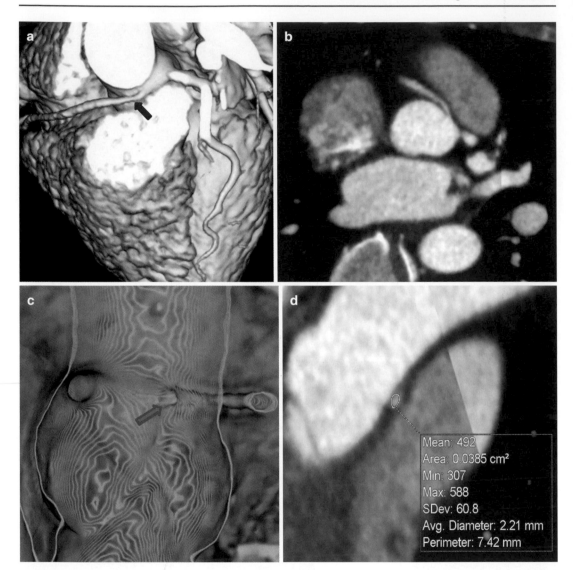

Fig. 3.23 (**a**) Volume rendered cranial anterior oblique image of the heart demonstrates an anomalous right coronary artery origin from the left Sinus of Valsalva (*black arrow*) with an aberrant retro pulmonic, pre aortic course. (**b**) Axial maximum intensity projection (MIP) image at the level of the Sinus of Valsalva demonstrates a 50 % diameter stenosis at the origin of the anomalous right coronary artery. (**c**) Volume rendered hollow projection image of inside the Sinuses of Valsalva demonstrates a small ostium of the right coronary artery (*blue arrow*) relative to the left. The right coronary artery ostium is anomalously located within the left Sinus of Valsalva. (**d**) Oblique multiplanar reformat of the aortic root in long axis demonstrates a moderately narrowed proximal RCA en face

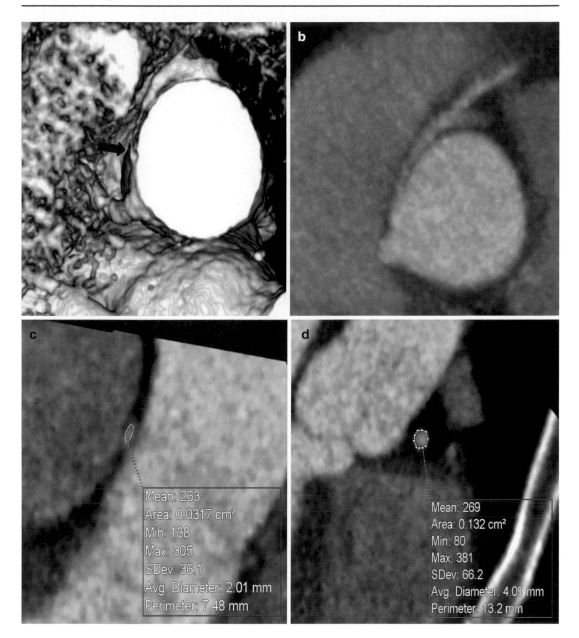

Fig. 3.24 (a) Volume rendered axial image at the level of the Sinus of Valsalva demonstrates an anomalous right coronary artery origin from the left Sinus of Valsalva (*black arrow*) with an aberrant retro pulmonic, pre aortic course and moderate 50 % diameter stenosis. (b) Axial maximum intensity projection image at the level of the Sinus of Valsalva demonstrates an anomalous right coronary artery origin from the left Sinus of Valsalva with an aberrant retro pulmonic, pre aortic course and moderate 50 % diameter stenosis. (c) Oblique multiplanar reformat of the aortic root in long axis demonstrates a 50 % diameter stenosis of the proximal RCA en face, with questionable intramural location. More distally (d) the RCA is normal caliber and within the epicardial adipose tissue

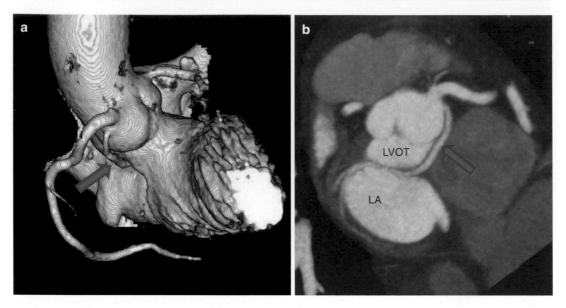

Fig. 3.25 (**a**) Volume rendered coronary image demonstrate anomalous origin of the RCA from right coronary cusp (*blue arrow*). (**b**) Oblique multiplanar reformat image shows anomalous LCX taking a retro aortic course between the left ventricular outflow tract (*LVOT*) and left atrium (*LA*) (*blue arrow*) finally emerging into the atrioventricular groove

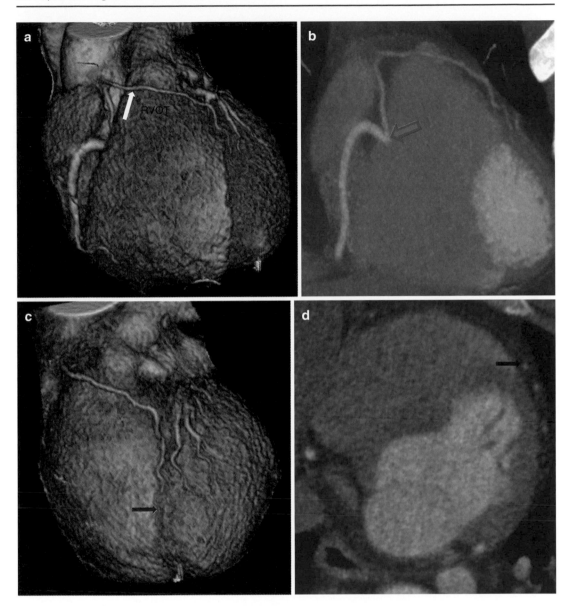

Fig. 3.26 (**a**, **b**) Coronal Volume rendered and maximum intensity projection image demonstrate anomalous origin of left anterior descending artery (*white arrow*) from proximal segment of right coronary artery (*blue arrow*). LAD courses anterior to the right ventricular outflow tract (*RVOT*). (**c**, **d**) Volume rendered and axial multiplanar images further demonstrating the course of anomalous LAD lying in the interventricular groove (*black arrow*) to the apex

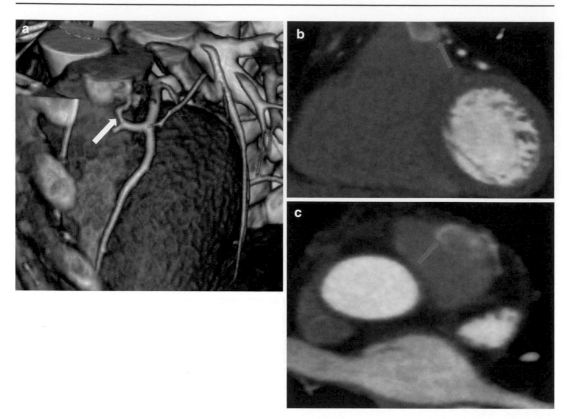

Fig. 3.27 (**a**) Volume rendered slightly oblique anterior (coronal) projection of the heart demonstrates a vessel originating from the mid LAD and coursing superiorly to enter the main pulmonary trunk (*white arrow*). (**b**) Oblique multiplanar reformatted near-coronal image of the heart demonstrates a small vessel with contrast entering the unopacified main pulmonary artery, resulting in a contrast blush (*blue arrow*). (**c**) Axial foot view image of the heart demonstrates a contrast blush in the main pulmonary artery consistent with left to right shunting of contrast from the LAD (*blue arrow*)

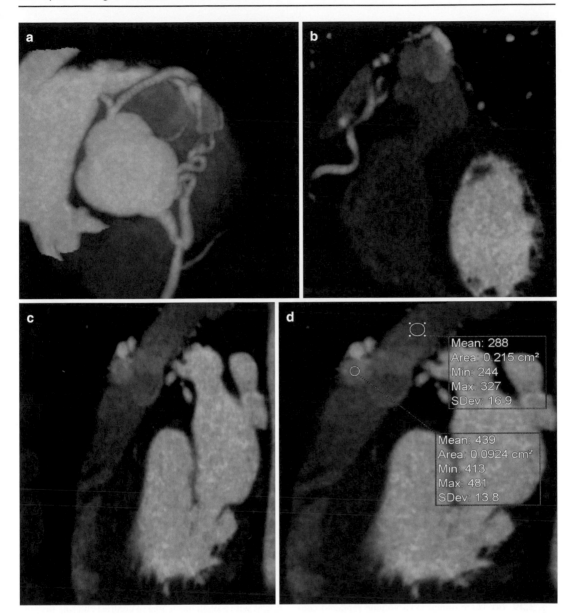

Fig. 3.28 (**a**) Oblique maximum intensity projection at the level of the Sinus of Valsalva demonstrates a tortuous vessel emanating from the left main coronary artery and extending toward the main pulmonary artery. (**b**) Near-coronal oblique MPR image through the RVOT and mid left ventricle demonstrates a tortuous dilated vessel cranial to the pulmonary valve, with a concomitant contrast blush within the unenhanced main pulmonary artery consistent with the left to right fistulous connection. (**c**, **d**) Near-sagittal right ventricular outflow tract (RVOT) image demonstrates contrast blush within the Sinus of Valsalva consistent with left to right flow from the high pressure LM to the low pressure main pulmonary artery. *Although visually apparent, Hounsfield Unit measurements may be useful in subtle cases. The HU prescribed here demonstrate a difference of over 10 standard deviations with regards to expected image noise*

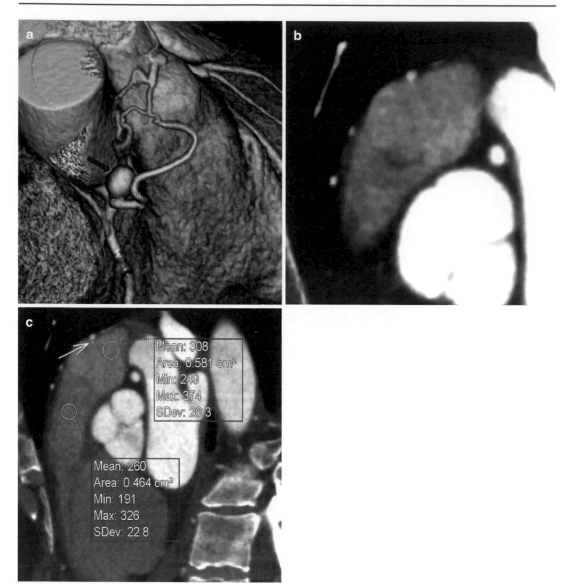

Fig. 3.29 (a) Three dimensional volume rendered caudally oriented, near anteroposterior projection image at the level of the aortopulmonary window demonstrates a prominent conus arteriosus branch emanating from the proximal RCA, coursing in its typical direction, but becoming focally aneurysmal (*black arrow*) before it enters the main pulmonary artery/trunk. (**b, c**) Oblique near axially oriented multiplanar reformat with the aortic valve en face demonstrates a prominent vessel intimately associated with the right wall of the main pulmonary artery, with a small linear area of contrast entering the pulmonary artery lumen (*arrow*). *As previously mentioned, HU determination may be useful to determine left to right shunting in patient with excellent contrast opacification of their left heart and excellent contrast nulling (via a saline chaser) of their right heart. Hounsfield Units in the main PA is two standard deviation above the unopacified blood pool in the RVOT consistent with a left to right shunt. Caution should be made when using this method as contrast admixture artifact may cause a false positive*

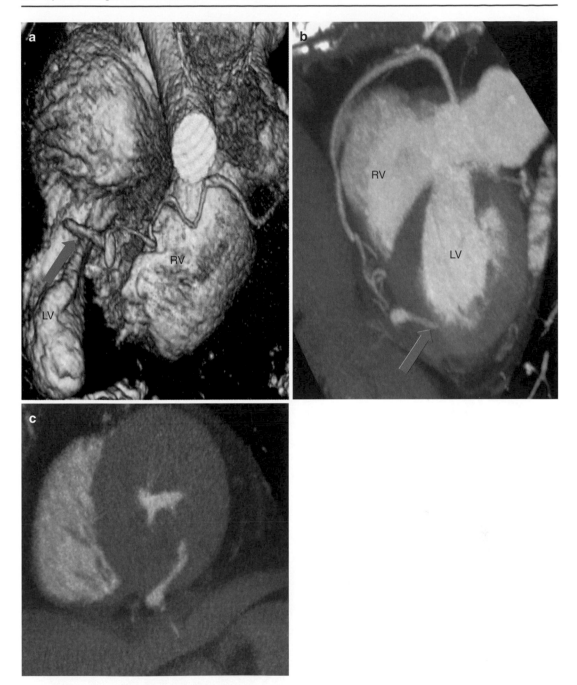

Fig. 3.30 (**a**) Volume rendered image demonstrate pooling of the contrast at the end of a vessel originating from distal RCA (*blue arrow*). (**b**) Near short-axis, LAO maximum intensity projection image at the level of the right Sinus of Valsalva demonstrates a tortuous vessel arising from distal RCA entering the inferior wall of the left ventricle with contrast seen within the myocardium and entering the blood pool. Consistent with fistulous connection between RCA and Left ventricle (*LV*). (**c**) Short axis at the mid-apex in systole demonstrates a tortuous vessel entering a contrast filled crevice within the inferior wall left ventricle. *As clearly seen the connection is not obvious in these images acquired during end systole. It is important to diagnose fistulous connection on images during diastole. RV* right ventricle

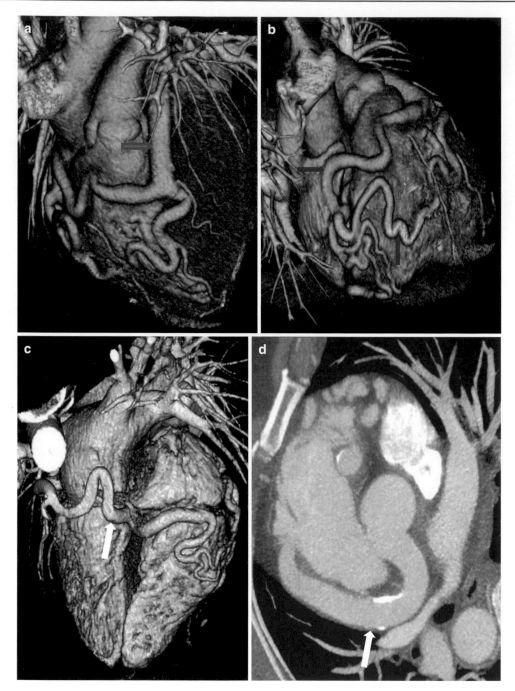

Fig. 3.31 (**a**, **b**) Volume rendered caudally oriented view of the heart demonstrates severely dilated LAD (*blue arrow*), Anomalous RCA, 2 branches from mid-LAD cross anterior to RV and supply RV (*red arrows*). (**c**) Dilated LCX courses in AV groove, supplies normal caliber LPL's then continues as dilated vessel across to RV (*white arrow*). (**d**) RV branches of the LAD and the distal LCX form confluence in the right AV groove that is calcified and aneurysmal (*white arrow*). (**e**) Distal to confluence, there is a common short segment artery with fistulous communication to the basal RV (superior to the tricuspid valve (*white arrow*). *Overall, this is a complex coronary AVF with distal LCX – LPLB and anomalous RCA feeding into a common aneurysmal confluence with then drainage into the basilar RV.* (**g**, **h**) The coronary artery to RV fistula has been coiled at the entry point to the RV (*white arrow*). The upper branch of the LAD to RV fistula has thrombosed at the level of the LAD bifurcation (*red arrow*). There is decreased filling of the lower branch of the LAD to RV fistula possibly due to presence of thrombus or decreased contrast opacification. No evidence of left to right intracardiac shunt

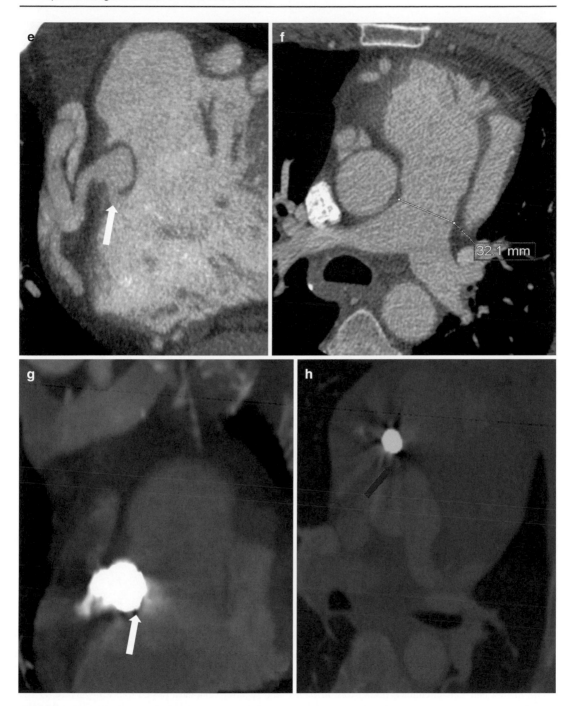

Fig. 3.31 (continued)

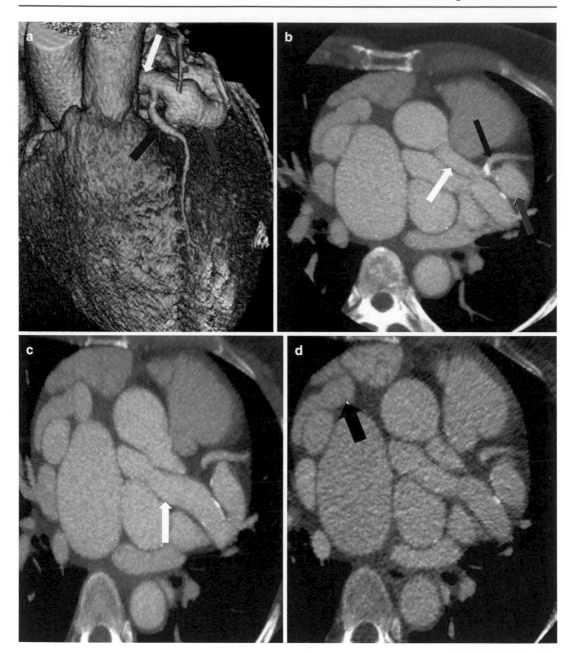

Fig. 3.32 (**a**, **b**) Volume rendered and maximum intensity projection image demonstrate aneurysmal left main (*white arrow*) and Left circumflex (LCX) (*red arrow*). Also noted is aneurysmal proximal segment of LAD (*black arrow*) which then continues as a normal sized vessel in the atrioventricular groove. (**c**) Maximum intensity projection image demonstrate aberrant course of a convoluted LCX though the transverse sinus between aortic root and left atrium (*white arrow*), (**d**) multiplanar reformat image demonstrate fistulous connection between LCX and superior vena cava (SVC) (*black arrow*). (**e**, **f**) The coronary artery to SVC fistula has been coiled at the entry point to the SVC (*white arrow*) and origin of LCX (*red arrow*). *There is contrast filling of the LCX and SVC distal to the coil indicative of residual follow and an unsuccessful coiling.* Compare to the prior case of coiling

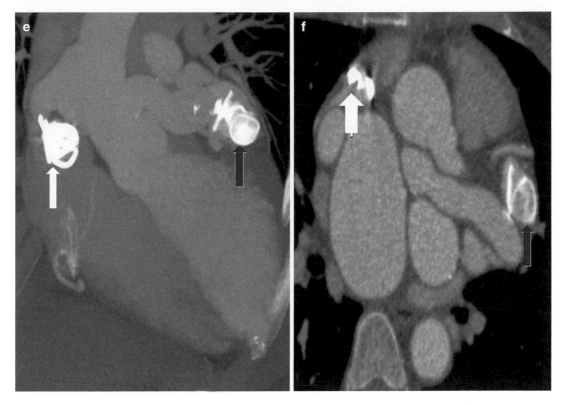

Fig. 3.32 (continued)

References

1. Leschka S, Oechslin E, Husmann L, et al. Pre- and postoperative evaluation of congenital heart disease in children and adults with 64-section CT. Radiographics. 2007;27:829–46.
2. Watts JR, Sonavane SK, Singh SP, et al. Pictorial review of multidetector CT imaging of the preoperative evaluation of congenital heart disease. Curr Probl Diagn Radiol. 2013;42:40–56.
3. Steiner RM, Reddy GP, Flicker S. Congenital cardiovascular disease in the adult patient. Imaging update. J Thorac Imaging. 2002;17:1–17.
4. Cook SC, Dyke PC, Raman SV. Management of adults with congenital heart disease with cardiovascular computed tomography. J Cardiovasc Comput Tomogr. 2008;2:12–22.
5. Samyn MM. A review of the complementary information available with cardiac magnetic resonance imaging and multi-slice computed tomography (CT) during the study of congenital heart disease. Int J Cardiovasc Imaging. 2004;20:569–78.
6. Anderson RH, Shirali G. Sequential segmental analysis. Ann Pediatr Cardiol. 2009;2:24–35.
7. Shinebourne EA, Macartney FJ, Anderson RH. Sequential chamber localization—logical approach to diagnosis in congenital heart disease. Br Heart J. 1976;38:327–40.
8. Carvalho JS, Ho SY, Shinebourne EA. Sequential segmental analysis in complex fetal cardiac abnormalities: a logical approach to diagnosis. Ultrasound Obstet Gynecol. 2005;26:105–11.
9. Webb GD, Mallhorn JF, Therrien J, Redington AN. Congenital heart disease. In: Bonow RO, Mann DL, Zipes DP, Libby P, editors. Braunwald's heart disease a textbook of cardiovascular medicine. 9th ed. Philadelphia: Elsevier; 2012. p. 1411–67.
10. Ritter DG, Seward JB, Moodie D, et al. Univentricular heart (common ventricle): preoperative diagnosis-hemodynamic, angiocardiographic and echocardiographic features. Herz. 1979;4:198–205.
11. Warnes CA, Liberthson R, Danielson GK, et al. Task Force 1: the changing profile of congenital heart disease in adult life. J Am Coll Cardiol. 2001;37:1161–98.
12. Moller JH, Taubert KA, Allen HD, Clark EB, Lauer RM, a Special Writing Group from the Task Force on Children and Youth, American Heart Association. Cardiovascular health and disease in children: current status. Circulation. 1994;89:923–30.
13. Reid GJ, Irvine MJ, McCrindle BW, et al. Prevalence and correlates of successful transfer from pediatric to adult health care among a cohort of young adults with complex congenital heart defects. Pediatrics. 2004; 113:e197–205.
14. Sommer RJ, Hijazi ZM, Rhodes Jr JF. Pathophysiology of congenital heart disease in the adult: part I: shunt lesions. Circulation. 2008;117:1090–9.
15. Marelli AJ, Mackie AS, Ionescu-Ittu R, et al. Congenital heart disease in the general population: changing prevalence and age distribution. Circulation. 2007;115:163–72.
16. Berko NS, Haramati LB. Simple cardiac shunts in adults. Semin Roentgenol. 2012;47:277–88.
17. Vogel M, Berger F, Kramer A, et al. Incidence of secondary pulmonary hypertension in adults with atrial septal or sinus venosus defects. Heart. 1999;82:130–3.
18. Gatzoulis MA, Freeman MA, Siu SC, et al. Atrial arrythmia after surgical closure of atrial septal defects in adults. N Engl J Med. 1999;340:839–46.
19. Brickner ME, Hillis LD, Lange RA. Congenital heart disease in adults. First of two parts. N Engl J Med. 2000;342:256–63.
20. Rouine-Rapp K, Russel IA, Foster E. Congenital heart disease in the adult. Int Anesthesiol Clin. 2012;50:16–39.
21. Calvert PA, Rana BS, Kydd AC, et al. Patent foramen ovale: anatomy, outcomes, and closure. Nat Rev Cardiol. 2011;8:148–60.
22. Homma S, Sacco RL. Contemporary reviews in cardiovascular medicine. Patent foramen ovale and stroke. Circulation. 2005;112:1063–72.
23. El-Chami MF, Hanna IR, Helmy T, Block PC. Atrial septal abnormalities and cryptogenic stroke: a paradoxical science. Am Heart Hosp J. 2005;3:99–104.
24. Knauth A, McCarthy KP, Webb S, Ho SY, Allwork SP, Cook AC, et al. Interatrial communication through the mouth of the coronary sinus. Cardiol Young. 2002; 12:364–72.
25. Quaife RA, Chen MY, Kim M, et al. Pre-procedural planning for percutaneous atrial septal defect closure: transesophageal echocardiography compared with cardiac computed tomographic angiography. J Cardiovasc Comput Tomogr. 2010;4:330–8.
26. Ko SF, Liang CD, Yip HK, et al. Amplatzer septal occluder closure of atrial septal defect: evaluation of transthoracic echocardiography, cardiac CT, and transesophageal echocardiography. Am J Roentgenol. 2009;193:1522–9.
27. Wan Y, He Z, Zhang L, et al. The anatomical study of left atrium diverticulum by multi-detector row CT. Surg Radiol Anat. 2009;31:191–8.
28. Abbara S, Mundo-Sagardia JA, Hoffmann I, Cury RC. Cardiac CT assessment of left atrial accessory appendages and diverticula. Am J Roentgenol. 2009; 193:807–12.
29. Peng LQ, Yu JQ, Yang ZG, et al. Left atrial diverticula in patients referred for radiofrequency ablation of atrial fibrillation. Assessment of prevalence and morphologic characteristics by dual-source computed tomography. Circ Arrhythm Electrophysiol. 2012;5:345–50.
30. Pochis WT, Saeian K, Sagar KB. Usefulness of transesophageal echocardiography in diagnosing lipomatous hypertrophy of the atrial septum with comparison to transthoracic echocardiography. Am J Cardiol. 1992;70:396–8.
31. Pharr JR, Figueredo VM. Lipomatous hypertrophy of the atrial septum and prominent crista terminalis appearing as a right atrial mass. Eur J Echocardiogr. 2002;3:159–61.
32. Nadra D, Nihoyannopoulos P. Lipomatous hypertrophy of the interatrial septum: a commonly misdiagnosed mass often leading to unnecessary cardiac surgery. Heart. 2004;99:e66.

33. Meaney JFM, Kazerooni EA, Jamadar DA, Korobkin M. CT appearance of lipmatous hypertrophy of the interatrial septum. AJR Am J Roentgenol. 1997; 168:1081–4.

34. Minette MS, Sahn DJ. Congenital heart disease for the adult cardiologist. Ventricular septal defects. Circulation. 2006;114:2190–7.

35. Warnes CA, Williams RG, Bashore TM, et al. ACC/AHA 2008 guidelines for the management of adults with congenital heart disease: A report of the American College of Cardiology/American Heart Association Task Force on Practice Guidelines (Writing Committee to Develop guidelines on the management of adults with congenital heart disease). Developed in collaboration with the American Society of Echocardiography, Heart Rhythm Society, International Society for Adult Congenital Heart Disease, Society for Cardiovascular Angiography and Interventions, and Society of Thoracic Surgeons. J Am Coll Cardiol. 2008;52:e1–121.

36. Feldman BJ, Khandheria BK, Warnes CA, et al. Incidence, description and functional assessment of isolated quadricuspid aortic valves. Am J Cardiol. 1990;65:937–8.

37. Olson LJ, Subramanian MB, Edwards WD. Surgical pathology of pure aortic insufficiency: a study of 225 cases. Mayo Clin Proc. 1984;59:835–41.

38. Timperley J, Milner R, Marshall AJ, Gilbert TJ. Quadricuspid aortic valves. Clin Cardiol. 2002; 25:548–52.

39. Hayes CJ, Gersony WM, Driscoll DJ, et al. Second natural history study of congenital heart defects: results of treatment of patients with pulmonary valvar stenosis. Circulation. 1993;87 Suppl 1:I-28–37.

40. Davia JE, Fenoglio JJ, DeCastro CM, McAllister HA, Cheitlin MD. Quadricuspid semilunar valves. Chest. 1977;72:186–9.

41. Fernández B, Fernández MC, Durán AC, et al. Anatomy and formation of congenital bicuspid and quadricuspid pulmonary valves in Syrian hamsters. Anat Rec. 1998;250:70–9.

42. Attenhofer Jost CH, Connolly HM, Dearani JA, Edwards WD, Danielson GK, Congenital Heart Disease for the Adult Cardiologist. Ebstein's anomaly. Circulation. 2007;115:277–85.

43. Kilner PJ. Imaging congenital heart disease. Br J Radiol. 2011;84:S258–68.

44. Celermajer DS, Bull C, Till JA, et al. Ebstein's anomaly: presentation and outcome from fetus to adult. J Am Coll Cardiol. 1994;23:170–6.

45. Schneider DJ, Moore JW. Patent ductus arteriosus. Circulation. 2006;114:1873–82.

46. Morgan-Hughes GJ, Marshall AJ, Roobottom C. Morphologic assessment of patent ductus arteriosus in adults using retrospectively ECGgated multidetector CT. AJR Am J Roentgenol. 2003;181:749–54.

47. Sebastia C, Quiroga S, Boye R, et al. Aortic stenosis: spectrum of diseases depicted at multisection CT. Radiographics. 2003;23(Spec Issue):S79–91.

48. Türkvatan A, Akdur PO, Ölçer T, Cumhur T. Coarctation of the aorta in adults: preoperative evaluation with multidetector CT angiography. Diagn Interv Radiol. 2009;15:269–74.

49. Haramati LB, Moche IE, Rivera VT, et al. Computed tomography of partial anomalous pulmonary venous connection in adults. J Comput Assist Tomogr. 2003; 27:743–9.

50. Dillman JR, Yarram SG, Hernandez RJ. Imaging of pulmonary venous developmental abnormalities. Am J Roentgenol. 2009;192:1272–85.

51. Demos TC, Posniak HV, Pierce KL, et al. Venous anomalies of the thorax. AJR Am J Roentgenol. 2004; 182:1139–50.

52. Cormier MG, Yedlicka JW, Gray RJ, Moncada R. Congenital anomalies of the superior vena cava: a CT study. Semin Roentgenol. 1989;24:77–83.

53. Powell AJ. Aortopulmonary collaterals in single-ventricle congenital heart disease. How much do they count? Circ Cardiovasc Imaging. 2009;2:171–3.

54. Boshoff D, Gewillig M. A review of the option for treatment of major aortopulmonary collateral arteries in the setting of tetralogy of Fallot with pulmonary atresia. Cardiol Young. 2006;16:212–20.

55. Prasad SK, Soukias N, Hornung T, et al. Role of magnetic resonance angiography in the diagnosis of major aortopulmonary collateral arteries and partial anomalous pulmonary venous drainage. Circulation. 2004; 109:207–14.

56. Brickner ME, Hillis LD, Lange RA. Congenital heart disease; second of two parts. N Engl J Med. 2000; 342:334–42.

57. Bertranou EG, Blackstone EH, Hazelrig JB, Turner ME, Kirklin JW. Life expectancy without surgery in tetralogy of Fallot. Am J Cardiol. 1978;42:458–66.

58. Murphy JG, Gersh BJ, Mair DD, et al. Long-term outcome in patients undergoing surgical repair of tetralogy of Fallot. N Engl J Med. 1993;329:593–9.

59. Dabizzi RP, Teodori G, Barletta GA, et al. Associated coronary and cardiac anomalies in the tetralogy of Fallot: an angiographic study. Eur Heart J. 1990; 11:692–704.

60. Gatzoulis MA, Munk MC, Merchant N, et al. Isolated congenital absence of the pericardium: clinical presentation, diagnosis, and management. Ann Thorac Surg. 2000;69:1209–15.

61. Garnier F, Eicher JC, Philip JL, et al. Congenital complete absence of the left pericardium: a rare cause of chest pain or pseudo-right heart overload. Clin Cardiol. 2009;3:E52–7.

62. Schiavone WA, O'Donnell JK. Congenital absence of the left portion of parietal pericardium demonstrated by nuclear magnetic resonance imaging. Am J Cardiol. 1985;55:1439–40.

63. Gassner I, Judmaier W, Fink C, et al. Diagnosis of congenital pericardial defects, including a pathognomic sign for dangerous apical ventricular herniation, on magnetic resonance imaging. Br Heart J. 1995; 74:60–6.

Coronary Artery Disease Evaluation Using Cardiac CTA

4

Muzammil H. Musani, Alan Vainrib, Rajesh Gupta, and Michael Poon

4.1 Introduction

The application of cardiovascular CT imaging toward the detection, characterization, and prognostication of coronary artery disease (CAD) is one of the most rapidly evolving and exciting aspects of cardiovascular medicine. Coronary computed tomographic angiography (CCTA) has revolutionized the diagnosis and management of coronary artery disease by providing new methods for noninvasive imaging of coronary arteries. Coronary arterial calcification of plaques, plaque progression, stenosis characterization, plaque analysis, and appropriate use criteria will be presented below.

4.2 Coronary Arterial Calcification

4.2.1 Background

Coronary arterial calcification (CAC) signifies the presence of coronary atherosclerosis and as a result is associated with increased risk of cardiovascular events. Although CAC has been noted both anatomically and pathologically for centuries, it was first associated with a worse

cardiovascular prognosis in the early 1980s using fluoroscopic imaging [1]. The emergence of electron beam CT(EBCT) revolutionized coronary calcium detection by providing the means for noninvasive detection and quantification. With improving spatial resolution and increased versatility, multidetector row CT scanners (MDCT) have replaced EBCT for the detection of coronary calcium. Using a standard method to quantify coronary calcification, this technology has provided a means for risk stratification beyond traditional Framingham risk factors.

4.2.2 Coronary Calcium Score

The method of standardizing the amount of coronary calcium present in the heart was devised by Arthur Agatston in the late 1980s. This technique uses a scoring system based on the peak density of calcium in a lesion, measured in Hounsfield units(HUs). A score of 1 is assigned for 130–199 HU, 2 for 200–299 HU, 3 for 300–399 HU, and 4 for 400 HU and greater. This weighted score is then multiplied by the area of calcification in a lesion. The total score of all lesions, as well as total score of each artery, is then added together and presented. A number of studies have classified the degree of coronary calcification and plaque burden based on the following scale: 0 – No identifiable disease, 1 to 99 – Mild disease, 100 to 399 – Moderate disease, ≥400 – Severe disease.

Electronic supplementary material The online version of this chapter 10.1007/978-3-319-08168-7_4 contains supplementary material, which is available to authorized users.

4.2.3 Use in Risk Stratification

Calcium scoring provides both diagnostic and prognostic information. Although plaque calcification does not raise the risk for plaque rupture, higher calcium scores are associated with an increased plaque burden and consequently an increased risk for acute coronary syndrome (ACS). In 8,855 initially asymptomatic adults 30–76 years old (26 % women) who self-referred for EBT CAC screening, elevated CAC was associated with an increased risk of coronary events at 37-month follow up (RR = 10.5, $P<0.001$), above traditional risk factors of diabetes and smoking, especially in women [2].

Calcium scoring is associated with coronary arterial stenosis. Numerous studies looking at asymptomatic and symptomatic individuals have shown that CAC scoring is sensitive but not specific in predicting a >50 % stenosis on angiography. A 2000 ACC/AHA consensus statement presented data from 16 studies, approximating the sensitivity and specificity of EBCT at 91 and 49 %, respectively [3]. Additionally, the ACCURACY trial showed that the sensitivity and specificity for CAC >0, >100, and >400 were 98 and 42, 88 and 71, and 60 and 88 %, respectively.

Calcium scoring additionally has been shown to independently add prognostic information regarding CHD events and mortality to traditional Framingham risk factors, regardless of ethnicity [4, 5]. Calcium scoring additionally improves risk classification and information provided from the MESA cohort [6]. Risk classification is most improved in patients at intermediate risk based on Framingham data. In accordance with this, a consensus 2007 document from AHA/ACCF regarding calcium scoring suggests CAC for cardiovascular risk assessment in selected asymptomatic adults at intermediate risk (10–20 %, 10-year risk) by the Framingham risk score and modified Framingham/ATP risk scores when it is expected to change management if reclassified to a high or low risk group.

Despite an association with increased cardiovascular events, there is no evidence to date that suggests that pharmacological risk factor modification in asymptomatic patients with elevated CAC improves outcomes [7].

4.2.4 How High CAC Affects Interpretation of CTA

The size of a coronary calcification may be overestimated due to the partial volume effect, otherwise known as "blooming artifact." This occurs when voxels surrounding a calcification that are only partially filled with calcification are mistakenly identified as having a higher attenuation value. This leads to an increased number of high attenuation voxels associated with a calcification and can consequently cause difficulty with the visualization of the coronary lumen [8]. Broadening the window level by increasing the window width, or similar to using bone window, can minimize blooming artifact and can improve the diagnostic value of CCTA. Despite this, it has been noted that the specificity is reduced in the presence of coronary artery calcium (86 versus 53 % for detection of $\geq$50 % stenosis with Agatston scores $\leq$400 versus >400) [9].

4.3 Types of Plaques

Plaques may be characterized based on their typical appearance. Intravenous contrast within an arterial lumen typically have attenuation coefficients between 200 and 400 Hounsfield units(HU). Structures outside the lumen that have lower attenuation than the lumen or are calcified are considered to be plaque. There are three main types of plaques: calcified, noncalcified, or partially calcified (mixed) [10]. Spotty calcification, a type of partial calcification associated with increased risk of rupture, has been defined as plaque with calcification less than 3 mm in size on curved multiplanar reformation images and occupying only one side on cross-sectional images [11].

4.4 Plaque Progression

Pathological observation has well delineated the mechanisms of progression of coronary plaque. Coronary arterial plaques begin with intimal thickening and xanthoma formation, then develop into fibrous-cap fibroatheromas, progress to thin-cap atheromas, and eventually undergo plaque rupture or erosion [12]. This progression is driven by inflammation. LDL is oxidized, promoting chemoattraction of macrophages that ultimately cause accumulation of cholesterol esters and free cholesterol. These lipid-laden macrophages then undergo apoptosis which leads to the formation and expansion of a necrotic plaque core. Poor clearance of necrotic cells increases plaque size, as well as intraplaque hemorrhage, and plaque healing with fibrosis. Increases in lesion burden compromise the vessel lumen only when greater than 40 % of cross-sectional luminal narrowing occurs [13]. Prior to this, plaques undergo a compensatory outward enlargement called positive remodeling (PR). Prior studies have defined PR as a change in the vessel diameter at a plaque site in comparison to the reference segment in normal-appearing vessel tissue proximal to the lesion. PR has been associated with increased risk of ACS [14]. Ultimately, repeated plaque rupture and progression leads to encroachment into the vessel wall considered negative remodeling (NR).

4.5 Degree of Stenosis

In comparison to quantitative invasive coronary angiography (QCA), CCTA predicts luminal stenosis with an accuracy of ±25 % [15]. Although tools for digital quantitative analysis of the degree of luminal stenosis, area stenosis, and plaque extent are available, their use has not improved interpretation precision. Consequently, the society for cardiovascular computed tomography(SCCT) recommends reporting quantitative luminal stenosis severity in broad ranges, in addition to qualitative terms(e.g., mild, moderate, severe) [16]. Currently, two quantification ranges are in use:

0 Normal: Absence of plaque and no luminal stenosis
1 Minimal: Plaque with <25 % stenosis
2 Mild: 25–49 % stenosis
3 Moderate: 50–69 % stenosis
4 Severe: 70–99 % stenosis
5 Occluded

0 Normal: Absence of plaque and no luminal stenosis
1 Mild: Plaque with <39 % stenosis
2 Moderate: 40–69 % stenosis
3 Severe: 70–99 % stenosis
4 Occluded

Although CCTA is rather accurate in identifying coronary stenosis, one of its limitations is its inability to assess the physiological significance of lesions. However, combining 16-slice CCTA with SPECT myocardial perfusion imaging has been shown to improve sensitivity and specificity of coronary lesions(e.g., 84–96 % and 74–95 %, respectively) [17]. A more recent further comparison of CCTA and SPECT MPI performed in the CORE320 study showed that CCTA had superior sensitivity and specificity for detecting >50 and >70 % stenoses on a per patient and per vessel basis when compared to SPECT MPI. Invasive QCA was used as the gold standard comparison test. The results of the trial are shown below [18].

4.6 Plaque Analysis

CCTA has the unique ability to detect calcified and noncalcified coronary arterial plaque prior to the development of significant arterial luminal narrowing and clinical symptoms [19, 20]. An advantage of CCTA over conventional angiography is its ability to image the vessel wall and surrounding structures which can allow for detailed descriptions and characterizations of coronary plaques. Further, axial imagery, multiplanar reconstructions to the centerline of a vessel, as well as cross-sectional analysis allow for more in-depth plaque analysis. This has provided CCTA with the ability to detect plaques with characteristics associated with plaque rupture such as presence of thrombus, small residual lumen, greater plaque burden, and positive remodeling [21]. Other characteristics such as low plaque density and spotty calcification have been associated with increased risk of coronary events. Despite this, we do not yet have evidence to suggest changes in lifestyle and medical therapy can alter outcomes in patients who have plaques with these characteristics, and further study is warranted.

Efficacy of 320-slice CCTA and SPECT MPI CAD detection

	Sensitivity	Specificity	Positive predictive value	Negative predictive value
Per patient – 50 % stenosis				
CCTA	91 %	74 %	83 %	85 %
SPECT	62 %	67 %	73 %	55 %
Per patient – 70 % stenosis				
CCTA	94 %	60 %	55 %	92 %
SPECT	71 %	67 %	73 %	73 %

4.7   Cardiac CTA Post Revascularization

Revascularization in coronary artery disease is one of the most frequent medical procedures worldwide and can be performed with coronary artery bypass grafting or percutaneous stenting [22]. The follow-up evaluations of these procedures have typically been performed using conventional angiography. Advancements in coronary CTA technology allow noninvasive evaluations of coronary artery disease, graft and stent patency, as well as complications.

The advent of 64-slice MDCT and dual-source CT provides improved temporal and spatial resolution with reduction in both cardiac and respiratory motion allowing for accurate vessel analysis. Additionally, three-dimensional processing and advanced software reconstructions give physicians the ability to evaluate vessels in multiple planes and projections. Sensitivity and specificity values reach near 100 % for graft occlusion and high-grade stenosis [23]. This chapter will review coronary revascularization techniques, bypass graft anatomy, imaging protocols, as well as follow-up assessment of grafts and stents. Additionally, evaluation challenges, including artifacts and complications, will be briefly reviewed.

4.7.1   Coronary Artery Bypass Graft Surgery

Two main approaches for performing coronary artery bypass grafting include traditional on-pump surgery, which utilizes cardiopulmonary bypass and minimally invasive grafting through port access, and off-pump surgery without cardiopulmonary bypass [24]. Depending on the approach, different types of arterial and venous grafts can be used. Arterial grafts are preferred as they have better patency rates compared to venous grafts.

It is important for the physician interpreting the scan to know standard graft anatomy. Venous grafts are larger than native coronary arteries and arterial grafts and are less subjected to cardiac motion [22]. The left internal mammary artery is usually anastomosed to the left anterior descending artery (LAD), diagonals, and/or obtuse marginal branches. The standard connections of the right internal mammary artery graft are to the LAD, proximal right coronary artery, obtuse marginal branches, or diagonals. The great saphenous vein *(GSV)* and radial artery can be used as free grafts to any coronary artery as a single graft. The GSV is usually directly anastomosed to the aorta, while the radial artery is commonly attached to internal mammary grafts and less frequently to the aorta. The gastroepiploic artery is rarely used to revascularize the posterior descending artery or to extend a left internal mammary graft [24].

Long-term clinical outcome after surgery depends on patency of bypass grafts and progression of native coronary artery disease [23]. Coronary CTA provides an excellent noninvasive assessment of both. Imaging protocols to specifically assess grafts are similar to standard coronary CTA. One difference is that the scan requires a larger scan range to extend superiorly to include the origins of the internal mammary arteries or include the upper abdomen if a gastroepiploic graft was used [24]. With 64-MDCT, the scan duration and breath hold is approximately 15 s.

Bolus tracking of nonionic, iodinated, low-osmolar contrast is used for consistent results and homogenous opacification of the coronary arteries. Typically, an amount of approximately 60–100 ml of contrast followed by a saline flush is sufficient for bypass imaging using 64-MDCT [24]. Beta-adrenergic medications are used to maintain a heart rate <70 beats per second. In a case of a slow and stable heart rate, prospective ECG triggering is preferred as it can reduce radiation dose by up to 90 % [24]. Retrospective ECG gating is essential in cases of heart rate instability to obtain images in evenly spaced phases of the cardiac cycle [23]. Slice thickness and reconstruction field of view should be as small as possible.

Assessment of bypass grafts involves the identification of a homogeneous, contrast-enhanced graft lumen and graft wall that has a regular shape and border [23]. Analysis of the graft is usually divided into three segments, the origin or proximal anastomosis of the graft, the body of the graft, and the distal anastomosis. In cases where the distal anastomosis is not well evaluated, it is considered patent if contrast is identified within the graft lumen [23].

Prior reports utilizing electron beam CT (EBCT) have found that high-grade stenoses in venous grafts are located along the body of the graft and not in the region of the distal anastomosis [22]. It has been reported that detection of graft occlusion is difficult in venous grafts with the right coronary artery as the recipient vessel. Recipient vessel location influences graft survival. Grafts to the left anterior descending artery and a native vessel diameter >2 mm have the best survival [22].

Some challenges to bypass graft imaging include small vessel diameter, metal clip artifacts, and cardiac motion; however, the advanced 64-MDCT scanners can mitigate these challenges due to rapid acquisition times and increased spatial resolution [22]. The imager should be aware of bypass graft complications, which include graft thrombosis, malposition, vasospasm, and aneurysm. Within 1 month after surgery, throm-bosis is the most common cause of graft failure and is due to platelet dysfunction at the site of endothelial damage related to surgical harvesting and anastomosis. After 1 year, atherosclerosis results in graft stenosis and occlusion; however, late IMA graft failure is usually due to disease progression in the native vessel distal to the anas-tomosis [23].

Coronary CTA can identify occluded grafts by nonvisualization of the graft. Other signs include a small outpouching of the most proximal part of an occluded graft from the ascending aorta as contrast may still fill the graft proximally. Also, part of an occluded graft may be visualized as a "ghost" [23]. The noninvasive evaluation of graft patency and native coronary artery disease progression is becoming more common due to advancements of CT scanner technology leading to increased accuracy, fast image acquisitions, and convenience of coronary vessel analysis.

4.7.2   Coronary Stents

The majority of coronary revascularization interventions involve placement of a coronary artery stent to provide scaffolding of the vessel wall [22]. There are substantial differences in the appearance of various stents on coronary CTA due to stent material, design, coating, and drug-eluting properties [25]. Many factors influence in-stent restenosis and thrombosis rates such as design, clinical scenario during placement, coronary anatomy, specific lesion morphology, and anticoagulant drugs [22].

Coronary stent sizes range from 2.5 to 5 mm and are chosen based on the diameter of the artery being treated. Most stents are made of metal struts and appear differently on CT based on strut material, design, and size. For example, visibility of the lumen is superior with magnesium struts compared with tantalum-coated stents. Additionally, drug-eluting stents are covered with polymer which stores the drug to be released within the first 2 months of implantation [25].

There are specific challenges involved with CT imaging of coronary stents. Technical issues include blooming artifacts due to beam hardening and partial volume effect, motion artifacts, geometric effects due to anatomy, and intravascular contrast enhancement. Beam hardening occurs when dense structures, like metallic material, rapidly absorb lower-energy photons of the X-ray beam causing the beam to be more intense once it reaches the detector [26]. Higher-energy photons are less sensitive to soft tissue and iodine attenuation causing CT density in surrounding soft tissue to appear "darker" than it should, and black streaks may occur [25].

Blooming artifact causes an apparent increase in strut size, thereby artificially narrowing the stent lumen. It is affected by beam hardening but is mainly due to partial volume effects. These effects are influenced by the reconstruction algorithm. When two different densities are included within a voxel like part of a metallic stent and the lumen, the average density of the two are displayed. The high CT density values of metal cause the average to always be higher than body tissue; thus, the window-level settings in CT angiography will rather resemble the stent struts. Improving spatial resolution leads to smaller voxels and decreases volume effects. Even with 64-MDCT and its ability for thinner slices and dedicated reconstruction kernels, artificial narrowing is still considerable at about 30–40 % [25]. Considerations to reduce metal artifacts include stents with thinner struts and those made of low-density metal like magnesium or cobalt–chromium alloys. Additionally, increasing the kV can minimize metal artifacts by avoiding the photon starvation effect. However, this increases radiation exposure to the patient and should be limited [26].

The use of 64-MDCT has greatly reduced issues regarding motion artifacts. Geometric effects from angulation of the stent to the scan plane affect the visibility of the lumen. It has been described that the lumen is best visible if the stent is positioned 0° or 90° to the z-axis; however, most coronary arteries course with angulation. Sufficient intravascular contrast enhancement, of more than 250 HU, is needed to counteract the negative effect of lower contrast-to-noise ratio from beam-hardening artifacts [26].

Imaging protocols must optimize temporal and spatial resolution given the specific challenges related to metallic stents. The best possible temporal resolution is achieved by optimal heart rate and positioning in the scanner as it is best to be of slower heart rate and at the center of the scan field. The scanner's detector size will determine the thinnest possible slices and therefore the best spatial resolution. The smallest possible field of view is reconstructed for optimal coronary stent evaluation. Interpretation of coronary CTA for stent evaluation involves careful window-level settings [25].

Coronary CTA has evolved as a reliable tool for noninvasive detection of in-stent restenosis, stent thrombosis, and stent fractures. Although there are many potential applications, CT imaging of stents is considered clinically appropriate for risk assessment after revascularization in patients who were asymptomatic or have a history of left main coronary artery stenting and a stent diameter of 3 mm or more [26]. Continued advancements in CT technology, software reconstruction, and examination protocols will likely bring coronary CTA in the forefront as the primary diagnostic modality for revascularization evaluation.

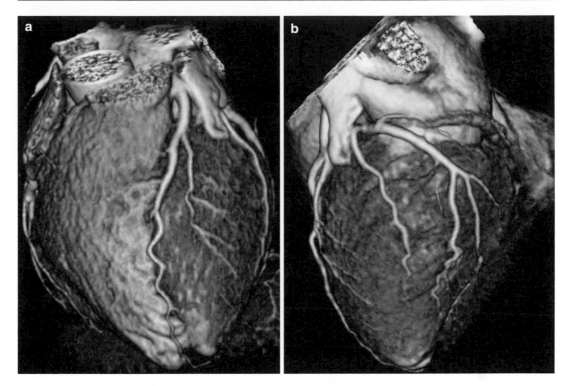

Fig. 4.1 (**a**) 3-dimensional volume rendered images of the heart demonstrating normal left anterior descending coronary arteries and its septal and diagonal branches. (**b**) 3D volume rendered images of the heart demonstrating normal left circumflex coronary artery and its obtuse marginal and posterolateral branches

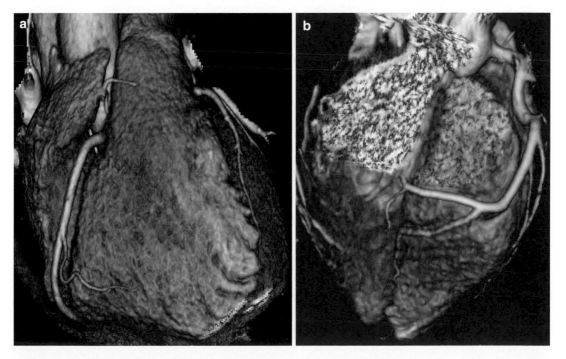

Fig. 4.2 (**a**, **b**) 3D volume rendered images demonstrating normal right coronary artery along with its branches conus, acute marginal and posterior descending arteries

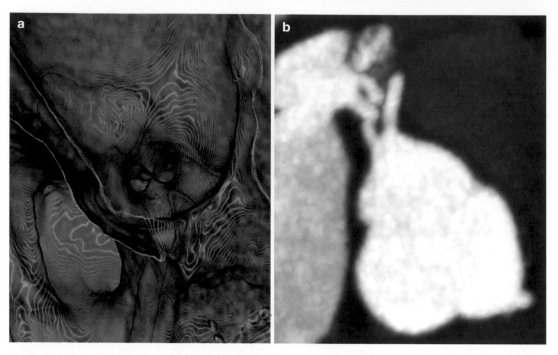

Fig. 4.3 (**a**) 3D Hollow volume rendered image from within the aorta demonstrating separate ostia of the LAD and LCX. (**b**) Multiplanar reformat image at the level of the aortic valve demonstrate separate ostia of the LAD and LCX from left coronary cusp

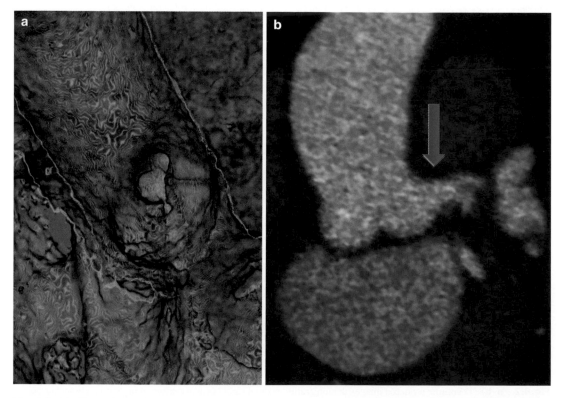

Fig. 4.4 (**a**) 3D hollow volume rendered image from within the aorta demonstrating a short left main (*blue arrow*) (compare to the prior image). (**b**) Multiplanar reformat image at the level of aortic valve demonstrating short left main originating from left coronary cusp

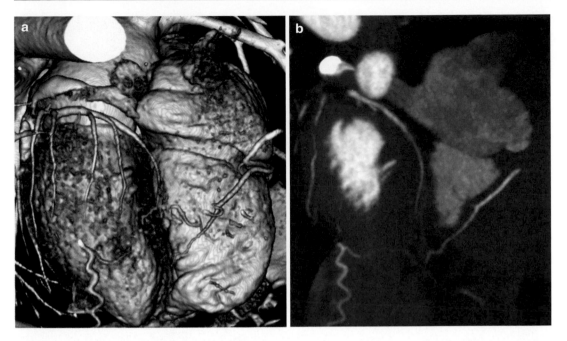

Fig. 4.5 (**a**) 3D volume rendered image demonstrating dual blood supply to the inferior wall coming from both LCX and RCA consistent with co-dominant circulation.

(**b**) Maximum intensity projection image demonstrating co-dominant circulation with left PDA and right PDA covering the inferior portion of the heart

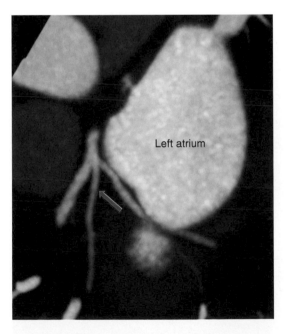

Fig. 4.6 Maximum intensity projection image demonstrating trifurcation of the LM into a prominent ramus intermedius branch (*blue arrow*), proximal LAD to the *left*, and proximal LCX to the *right*

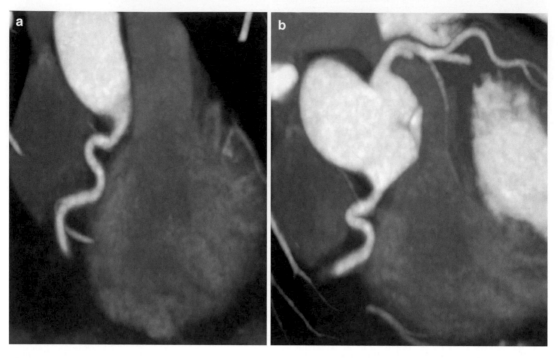

Fig. 4.7 (**a**, **b**) maximum intensity projection images demonstrating very tortuous proximal RCA and mid LAD resembling shepherd's crook

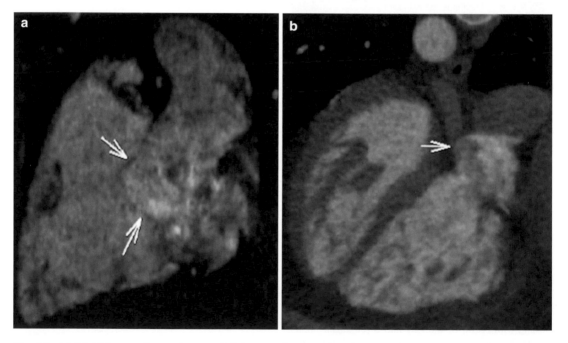

Fig. 4.8 (**a**) Multiplanar reformat image of right two chamber view demonstrating tricuspid valve (*arrow*). (**b**) Multiplanar reformat image demonstrating coronary sinus and thebesian valve (*arrow*)

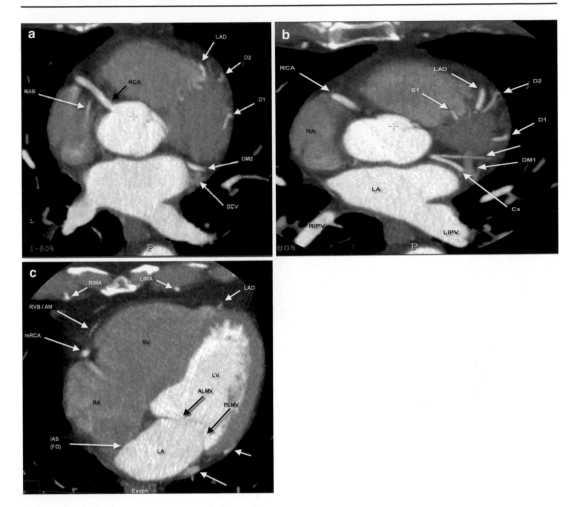

Fig. 4.9 (a) Axial MPR image demonstrating the following structures: *LAD* left anterior descending artery, *D1* 1st diagonal branch, *D2* 2nd diagonal branch, *OM2* 2nd obtuse marginal branch, *GCV* great cardiac vein, *RCA* right coronary artery, *RAB* right atrial branch. (b) Axial MPR image demonstrating following structures: *LAD* left anterior descending artery, *D1* 1st diagonal branch, *D2* 2nd diagonal branch. *S1* septal branch, *LCX* left circumflex artery, *OM1* 1st obtuse marginal branch, *GCV* great cardiac vein, *RCA* right coronary artery, *RA* right atrium, *LA* left atrium, *RIPV* right inferior pulmonary vein, *LIPV* left inferior pulmonary vein. (c) Four chamber MPR image demonstrating following structures: *LAD* left anterior descending artery, *OM* obtuse marginal branch, *RCA* right coronary artery, *RVB* right ventricular branch, *IAS* inter atrial septum, *LIMA* left Internal mammary artery, *RIMA* right internal mammary artery, *ALMV* anterior leaflet of the mitral valve, *PLMV* posterior leaflet of the mitral valve, *RV* right ventricle, *LV* left ventricle, *LA* left atrium, *RA* right Atrium

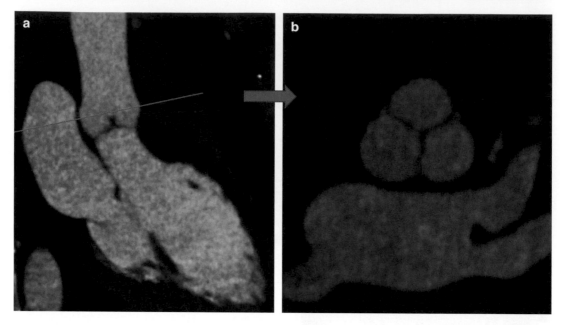

Fig. 4.10 (**a**) Three chamber/LV outflow tract view of the heart. *Blue line* depicts the level at which, Cross sectional view of the aortic valve is obtained 10 (**b**)

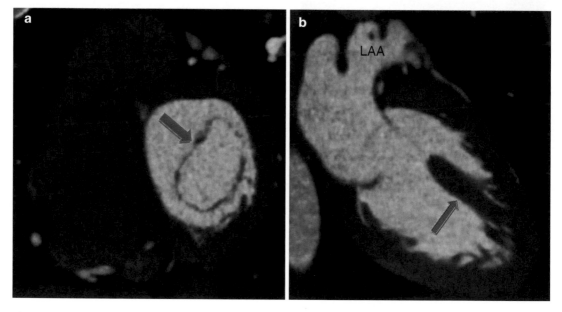

Fig. 4.11 (**a**) Short axis Multiplanar Reformat image at the level of the mitral valve leaflet (*arrow*). (**b**) Left Two chamber Multiplanar Reformat image demonstrating left atrial appendage (*LAA*) and anterolateral papillary muscle (*arrow*)

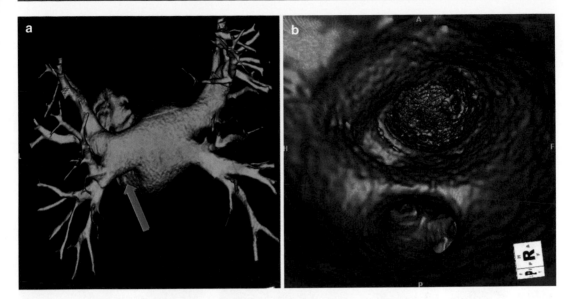

Fig. 4.12 (**a**) 3D volume rendered image of the left atrium and the associated pulmonary veins. A common left pulmonary vein trunk is noted (*arrow*). (**b**) Hollow 3D volume rendered image of the inside view of the ostia of the pulmonary veins

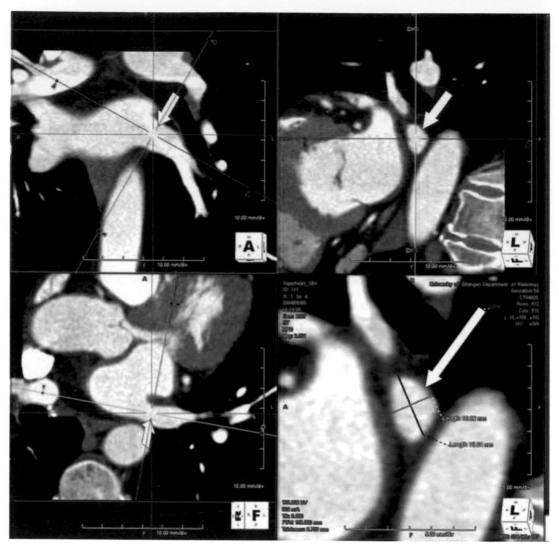

Fig. 4.13 Multiple multiplanar reformat images demonstrate how to obtain cross sectional measurements of each individual pulmonary veins important prior to atrial fibrillation ablation

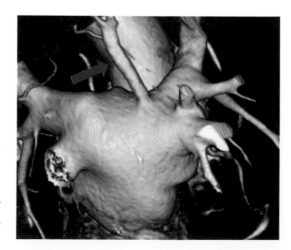

Fig. 4.14 3D volume rendered image demonstrate superior Accessory Pulmonary vein (*arrow*)

Fig. 4.15 3D volume rendered images demonstrate venous system of the heart. *GCV* great cardiac vein, *CS* coronary sinus, *PVLV* posterior vein of the left ventricle, *PIV* posterior interventricular vein, *LMV* left marginal vein, *RA* right atrium, *LA* left atrium, *RV* right ventricle, *LV* left ventricle

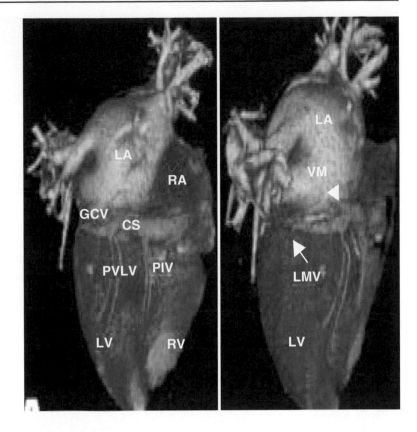

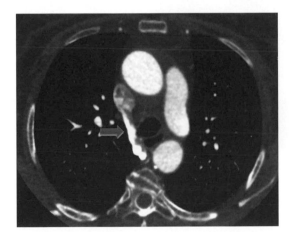

Fig. 4.16 Axial image demonstrate Azygous vein (*arrow*) draining into the superior vena cava

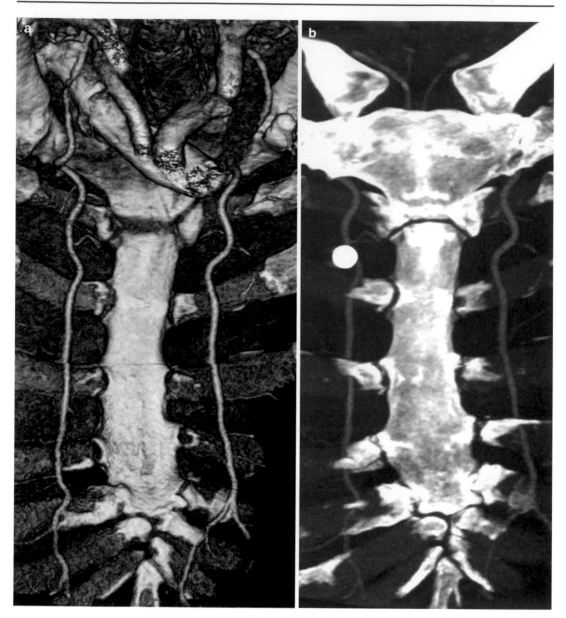

Fig. 4.17 (**a**, **b**) Posteroanterior 3D volume rendered and maximum intensity images demonstrating right and left internal mammary arteries. Also note blooming artifact from extensive calcification in left main, proximal LAD and proximal LCX limiting accurate assessment of luminal stenosis

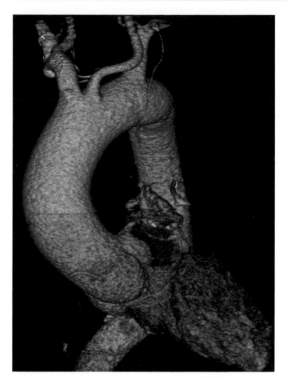

Fig. 4.18 3D volume rendered image of thoracic aorta with origin of right brachiocephalic truck, left common carotid and left subclavian artery

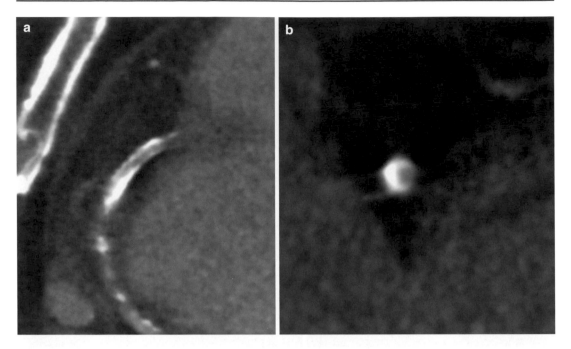

Fig. 4.24 (**a**) Multiplanar reformat contrast images of the right coronary artery demonstrate extensive calcification mimicking a stent in a longitudinal view. It is impor- tant to visualize cross section which in this case (**b**) demonstrate near circumferential calcification which is not evenly distributed

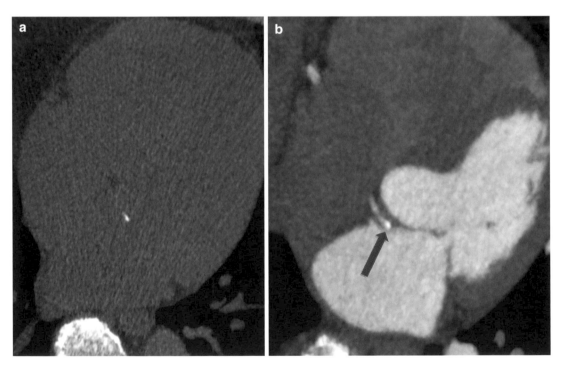

Fig. 4.25 (**a**) Axial multiplanar reformat noncontrast image demonstrate focal small calcification in a noncoro- nary distribution. (**b**) Axial multiplanar reformat contrast image demonstrate anomalous left circumflex with small focal calcified plaque (*arrow*)

It is important to identify cases in which viewing contrast images prior to calculating calcium score can play a crucial role

4.9   Nonobstructive Coronary Artery Disease

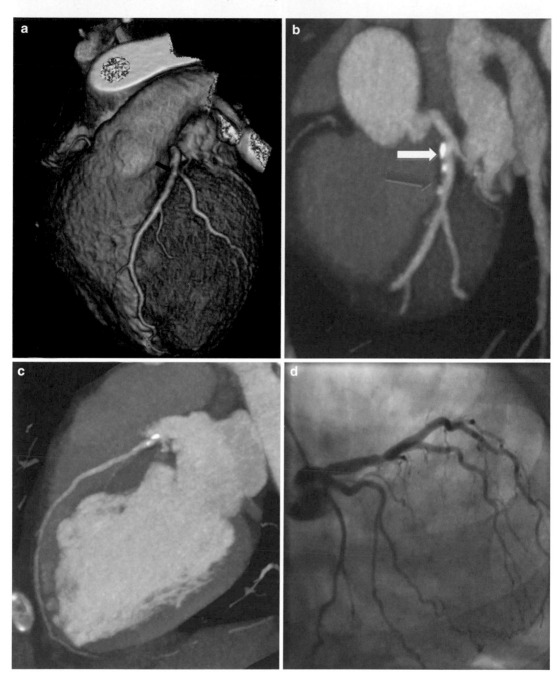

Fig. 4.26 (a) 3D volume rendered image demonstrate subtle bump of calcification in proximal and mid LAD (*black arrow*). (b) Maximum intensity projection image demonstrate nonobstructive calcified (*white arrow*) and partially calcified plaques (*blue arrow*) in proximal LAD. (c) Maximum intensity projection image in near two chamber view demonstrate nonobstructive calcified and partially calcified plaques in proximal and mid LAD. (d) Coronary angiographic correlation demonstrate atherosclerotic plaque causing mild stenosis. (e) Maximum intensity projection image demonstrating nonobstructive calcified plaque in proximal and mid RCA causing minimal stenosis. (f) Coronary angiography confirms CCTA findings

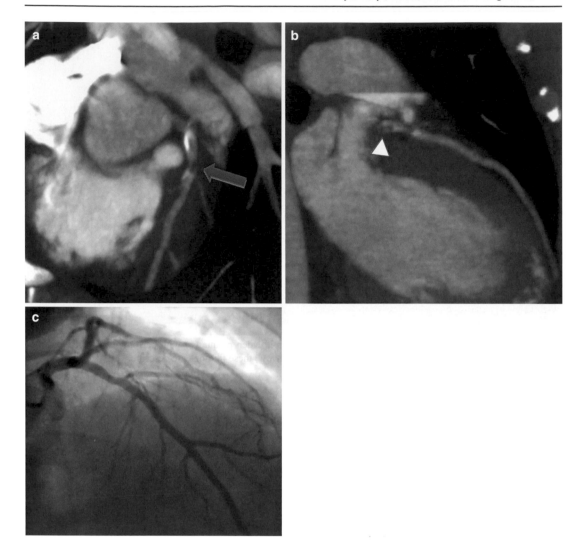

Fig. 4.28 (**a**, **b**) Maximum intensity projection images demonstrate obstructive calcified plaque in proximal LAD (*arrow*), please note significant motion artifact as indicated by blurring of the vessel wall (*arrow head*) compare to the distal vessel. (**c**) Coronary angiography in this patient revealed nonobstructive plaque in proximal to mid LAD

Note

Motion artifact is one of the most common reason for overestimating luminal stenosis and leading to false positive results. It is therefore important to assess the luminal stenosis in different phases of cardiac cycle

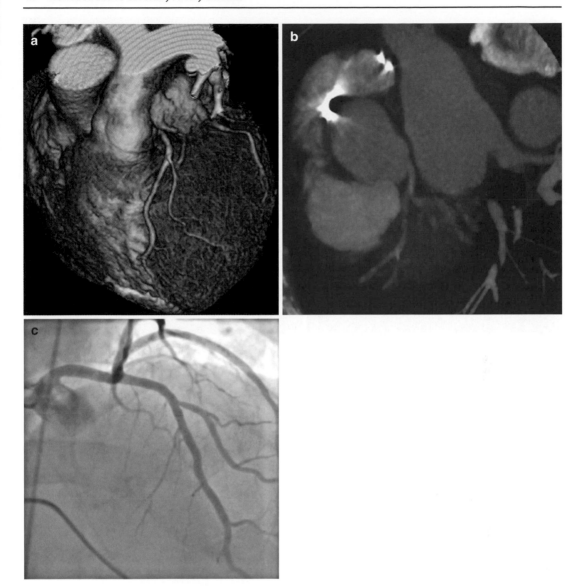

Fig. 4.29 (a) 3D volume rendered image demonstrate LAD no area of stenosis. (b) Maximum intensity projection image demonstrate significant motion artifact creating an impression of high grade stenosis patient was referred for cardiac catheterization. (c) Coronary angiographic correlation revealed normal appearing LAD

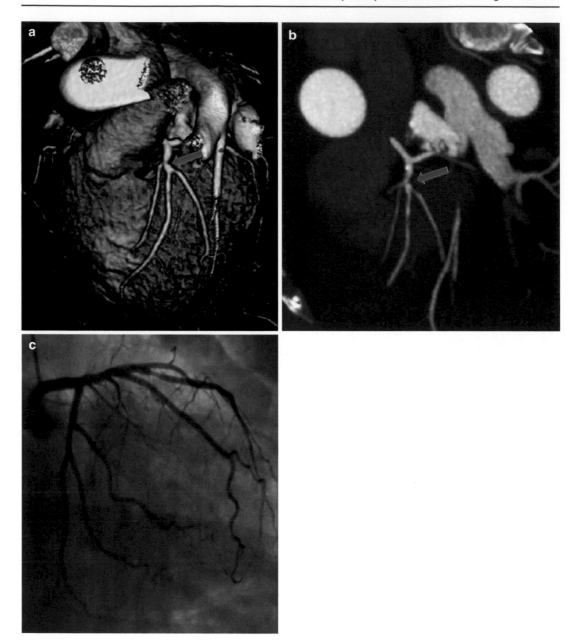

Fig. 4.30 (**a**) 3D volume rendered image demonstrate narrowing in proximal to mid lad (*arrow*). (**b**) Maximum intensity projection image demonstrate non obstructive partially calcified plaque in proximal to mid lad (*arrow*) with extension into ostium of 1st diagonal branch. (**c**) Coronary Angiographic correlation reveals nonobstructive plaque in proximal LAD and 1st diagonal branch

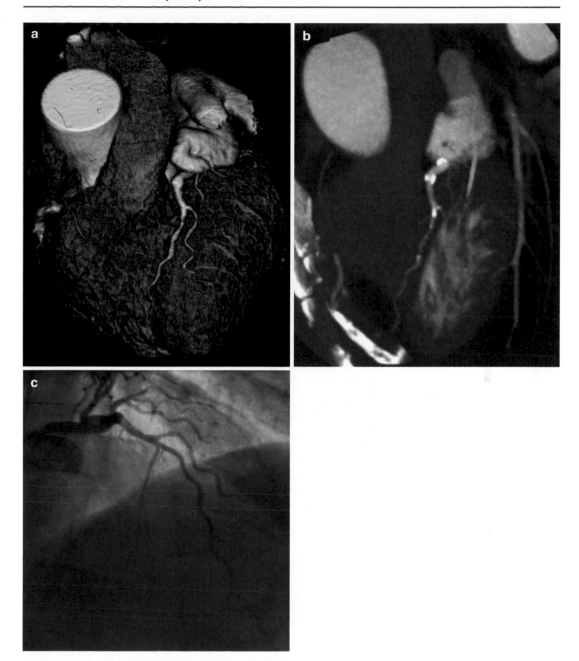

Fig. 4.31 (**a**) 3D volume rendered image demonstrate calcified plaque in proximal and mid LAD. (**b**) Demonstrate dense calcified plaque in proximal and mid LAD limiting accurate assessment of degree of luminal stenosis. (**c**) Coronary angiography demonstrate nonobstructive coronary artery disease in proximal and mid lad

Note

Dense calcification is one of the biggest limitations for cardiac CTA when it comes to coronary artery disease evaluation. It is also one of the most important factor for over estimating luminal stenosis. Please refer to chapter on artifacts for methods to minimize blooming from calcium and better assessment of luminal stenosis

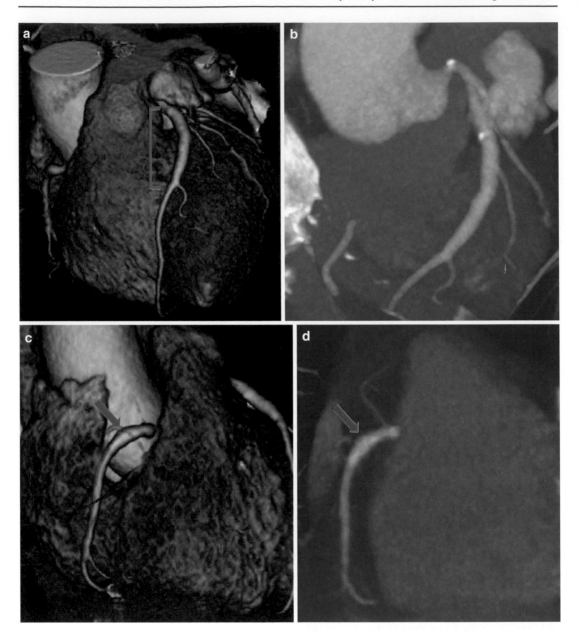

Fig. 4.32 (**a**) 3D volume rendered and maximum intensity projection image demonstrate ectatic proximal and mid LAD. (**b**) Also noted is calcified plaque in left main and mid LAD. (**c, d**) 3D volume rendered and maximum intensity projection images of the same patient demonstrate ectatic proximal RCA (*Blue arrow*)

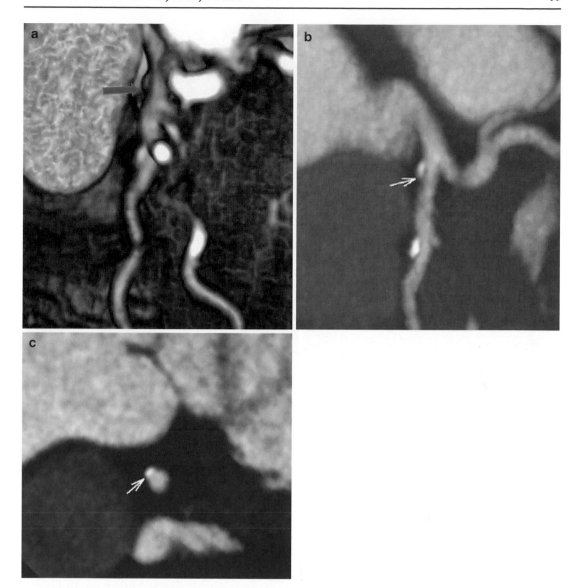

Fig. 4.33 (a) 3D volume rendered image demonstrate a bump in proximal LAD (*blue arrow*), (b) maximum intensity projection image demonstrate calcified plaque in proximal LAD with outward extension and no luminal compromise suggestive of positive remodelling (*arrow*). (c) Cross sectional of the vessel clearly demonstrate the phenomenon of positive remodelling (*arrow*)

4.10   Obstructive Coronary Artery Disease

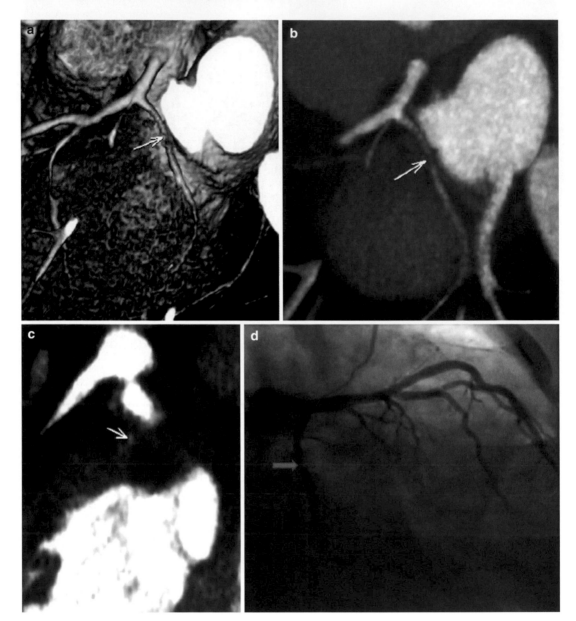

Fig. 4.34 (**a**) 3D volume rendered image demonstrate significant luminal narrowing in proximal left circumflex (*arrow*). (**b**) Maximum intensity projection image demonstrate obstructive noncalcified plaque proximal left circumflex (*arrow*) with poor contrast flow distally. (**c**) Cross sectional multiplanar reformat image of proximal left circumflex demonstrating obstructive noncalcified plaque (*arrow*). (**d**) Coronary angiographic correlation reveals high grade stenosis in proximal left circumflex (*arrow*) (Video 4.1)

Patient was a 38 -year old male with zero calcium score presenting to the ED with complains of Chest pain

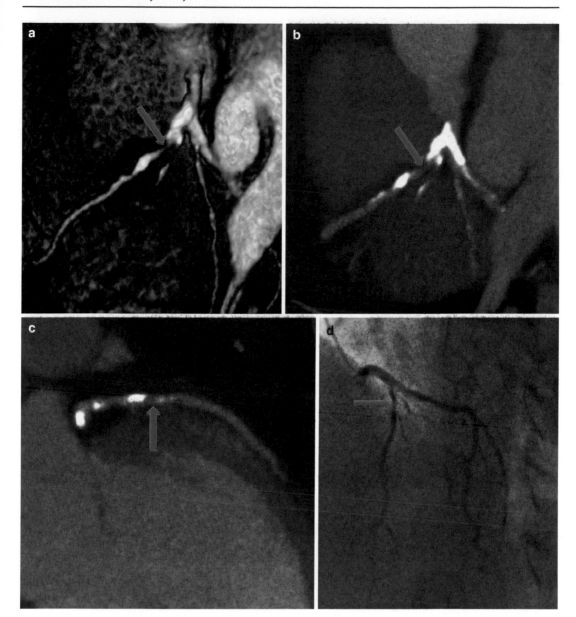

Fig. 4.35 (**a**) 3D volume rendered image demonstrate significant luminal narrowing in mid LAD (*arrow*). (**b**) Maximum intensity projection image demonstrate obstructive partially calcified plaque in mid LAD (*arrow*). (**c**) Maximum intensity projection image of LAD in longi-tudinal view demonstrating obstructive plaque in a different view (*arrow*). (**d**) Coronary angiographic correlation reveals high grade stenosis in mid LAD (*arrow*). (**e**) Fractional Flow Reserve across the mid LAD lesion has an FFR of 0.80

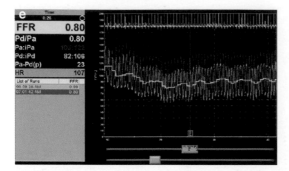

Fig. 4.35 (continued)

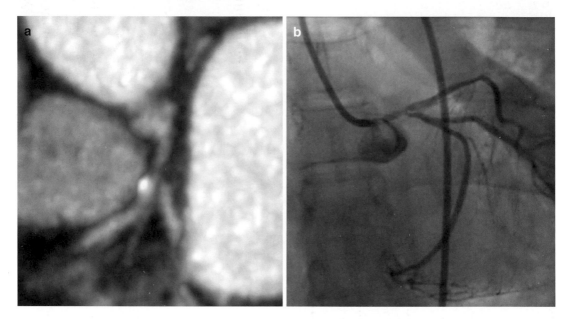

Fig. 4.36 (**a**) Multiplanar reformat image demonstrate obstructive partially calcified plaque extending from distal left main into proximal LAD and LCX. (**b**) Coronary Angiographic correlation confirms CCTA findings (Video 4.2)

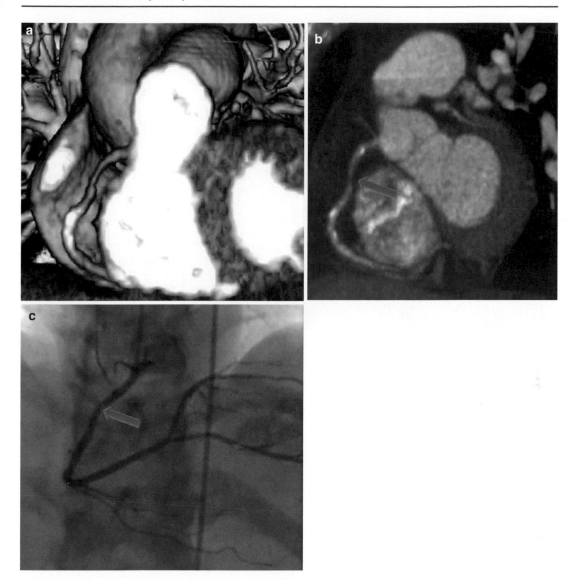

Fig. 4.37 (**a**) 3D volume rendered image demonstrate significant luminal narrowing of proximal RCA. (**b**) Maximum intensity projection image demonstrate obstructive partially calcified plaque in proximal RCA (*arrow*). (**c**) Coronary angiography confirms CCTA findings (*arrow*)

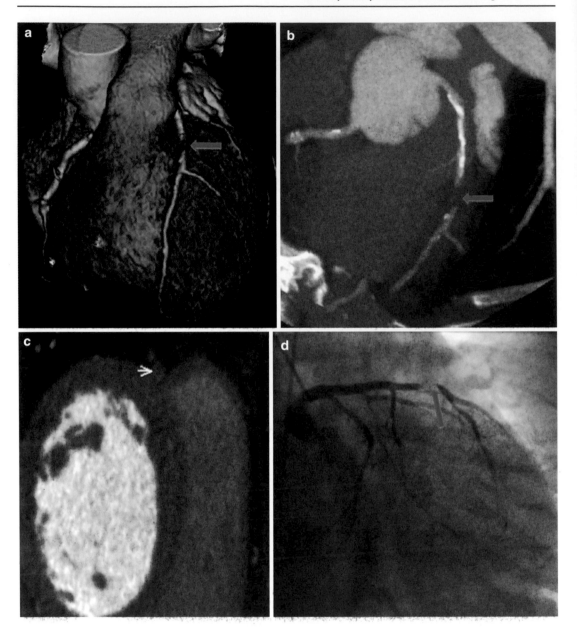

Fig. 4.38 (a) 3D volume rendered image demonstrate total occlusion (*arrow*) of mid LAD. (b) Maximum intensity projection image demonstrate total occlusion of mid LAD (*arrow*), also noted are nonobstructive calcified plaque in left main, proximal and mid LAD. (c) Cross sectional multiplanar reformat image demonstrates totally occluded segment of mid LAD (*white arrow*). (d) Coronary angiography demonstrate a high grade stenosis with a very small luminal patency (*arrow*)

Patient presented to the ED with complains of Chest pain and had positive troponins post CCTA

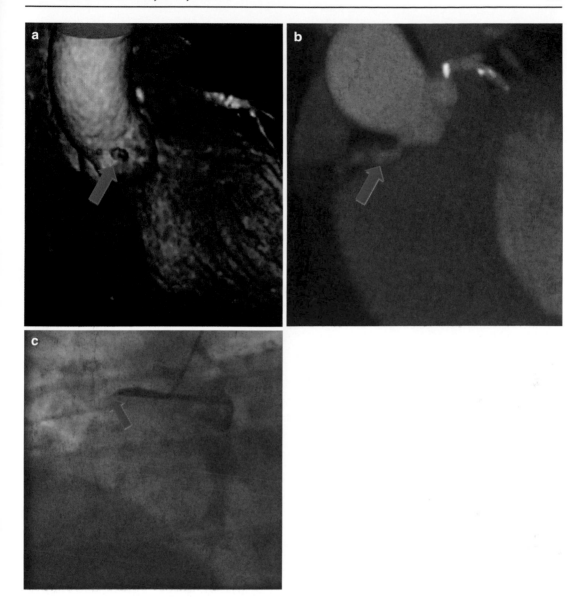

Fig. 4.39 (**a**) 3D volume rendered image demonstrate stump of proximal RCA (*arrow*) suggestive of total occlusion. (**b**) Multiplanar reformat image demonstrate total occlusion of proximal RCA (*arrow*). (**c**) Coronary angiograph confirms occluded proximal RCA (Video 4.3)

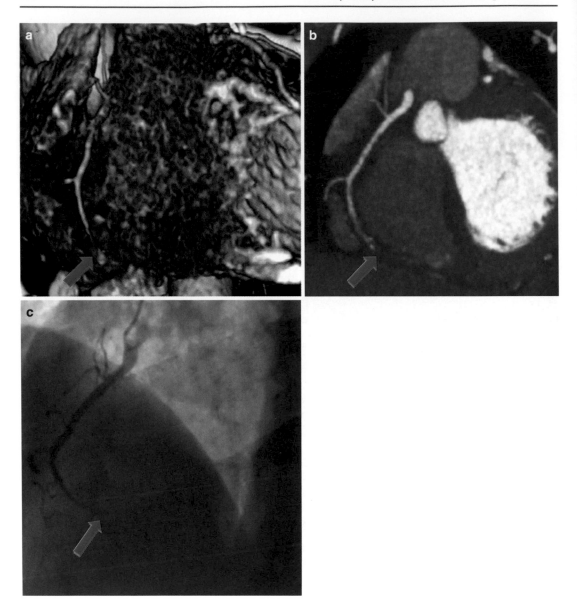

Fig. 4.40 (**a**) 3D volume rendered image demonstrate totally occluded distal RCA (*arrow*). (**b**) Maximum intensity projection image demonstrate total occlusion of distal RCA (*arrow*). (**c**) Coronary angiography confirms CCTA findings of occluded distal RCA (Video 4.4)

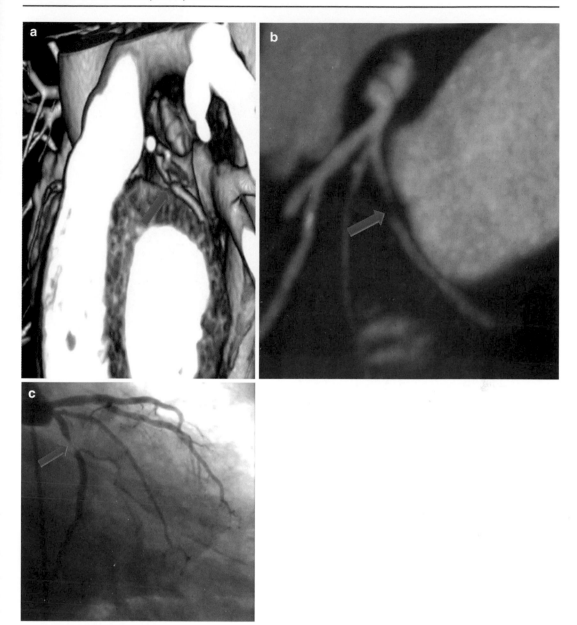

Fig. 4.41 (**a**, **b**) 3D volume rendered and maximum intensity projection images demonstrate obstructive noncalcified plaque in mid LCX (*blue arrow*). (**c**) Coronary angiography demonstrate confirms CCTA findings (*arrow*) (Video 4.5)

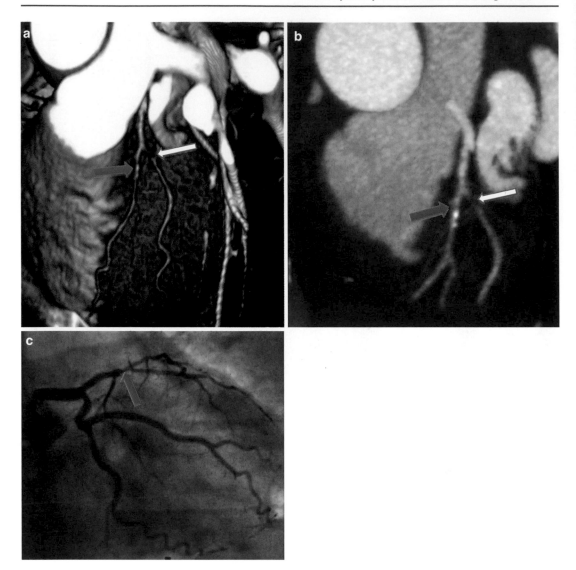

Fig. 4.42 (**a**, **b**) 3D volume rendered and maximum intensity projection images demonstrate obstructive partially calcified plaque in mid lad (*blue arrow*) and obstructive noncalcified plaque in 1st diagonal branch. (**c**) Coronary angiography confirms the CCTA findings (*arrow*) (Video 4.6)

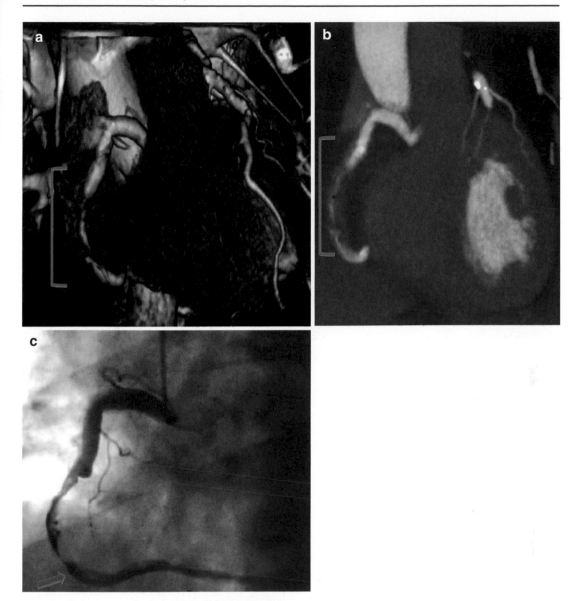

Fig. 4.43 (**a**) 3D volume rendered image demonstrate luminal irregularity in mid RCA. (**b**) Maximum intensity projection image demonstrate contrast streaking (*) through thrombus in mid RCA. (**c**) Coronary angiographic correlation reveals acute thrombus in mid to distal RCA with contrast pooling (*arrow*). Patient underwent thrombectomy along with 48 h of Hepranization prior to percutaneous coronary intervention (Video 4.7)

Diagnostic Pearls

CT images can be helpful in differentiating thrombus from plaque by measuring hounsfield units. Also thrombus appears to have appearance of luminal irregularities notes above

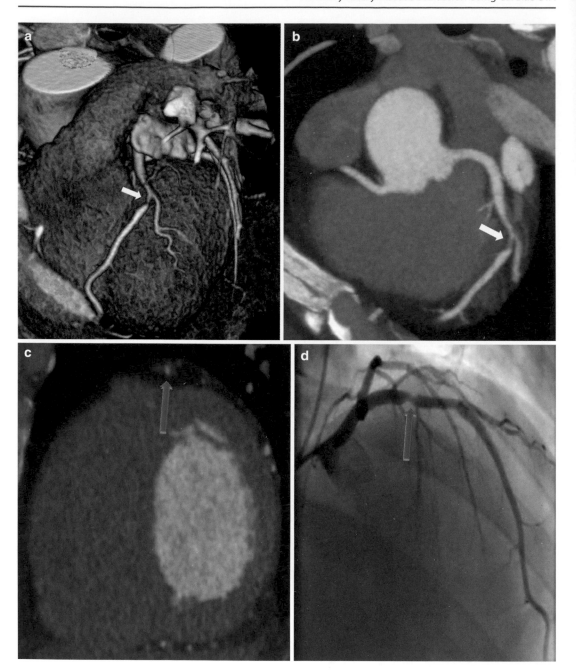

Fig. 4.44 (**a**) 3D volume rendered demonstrate significant luminal narrowing in proximal and mid LAD (*white arrow*). (**b**) Maximum intensity projection image demonstrate obstructive noncalcified plaque in proximal to mid LAD (*white arrow*). (**c**) Cross sectional multiplanar refor- mat image of mid lad demonstrating obstructive noncalcified plaque (*arrow*). (**d**) Coronary angiographic correlation reveals high grade stenosis in mid LAD (*arrow*) (Video 4.8)

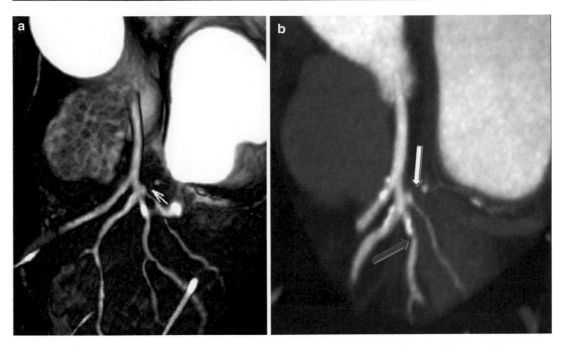

Fig. 4.45 (**a**, **b**) 3D volume rendered and maximum intensity projection demonstrate to totally occluded proximal left circumflex (*white arrow*). Also note obstructive partially calcified plaque in a large branching ramus branch (*blue arrow*)

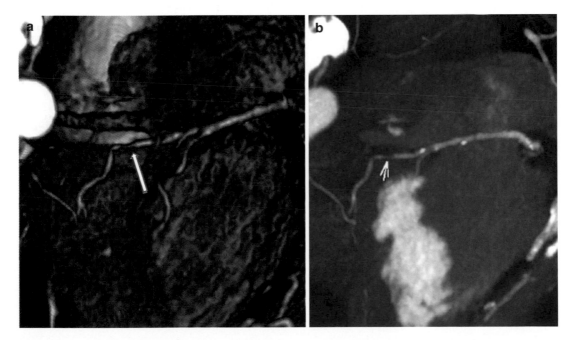

Fig. 4.46 (**a**) 3D volume rendered image demonstrate high grade stenosis in the right postero lateral (PL) branch (*arrow*). (**b**) Maximum intensity projection image demonstrate obstructive noncalcified plaque in right PL branch (*arrow*). Also note nonobstructive calcified plaque in distal RCA

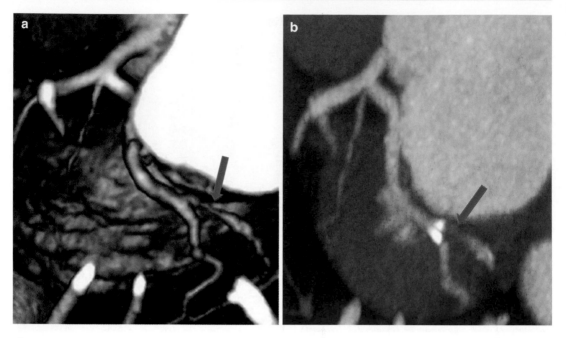

Fig. 4.47 (**a**) 3D volume rendered image demonstrate high grade stenosis in mid left circumflex (*arrow*). (**b**) Maximum intensity projection image demonstrate obstructive partially calcified plaque in mid LCX (*arrow*)

4.11   CCTA for Coronary Revascularization

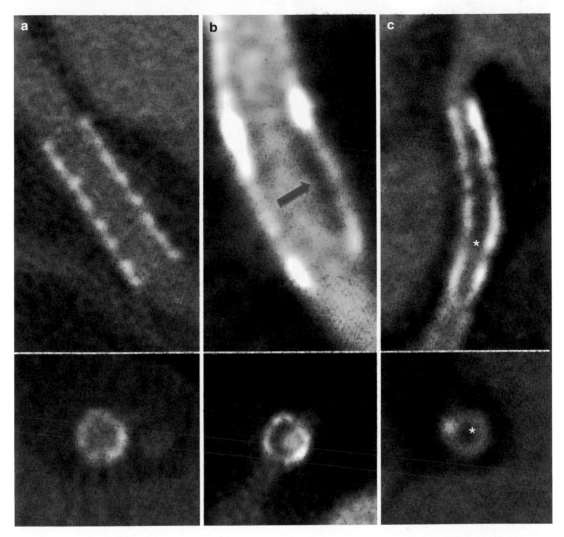

Fig. 4.48 (**a**) Multiplanar reformat longitudinal (*above*) and cross sectional image demonstrate patent stent in mid LAD. (**b**) Multiplanar reformat longitudinal and cross sectional image demonstrate patent stent with intimal hyperplasia (*arrow*). (**c**) Multiplanar reformat image demonstrate totally occluded stent no contrast appreciated in the lumen (*)

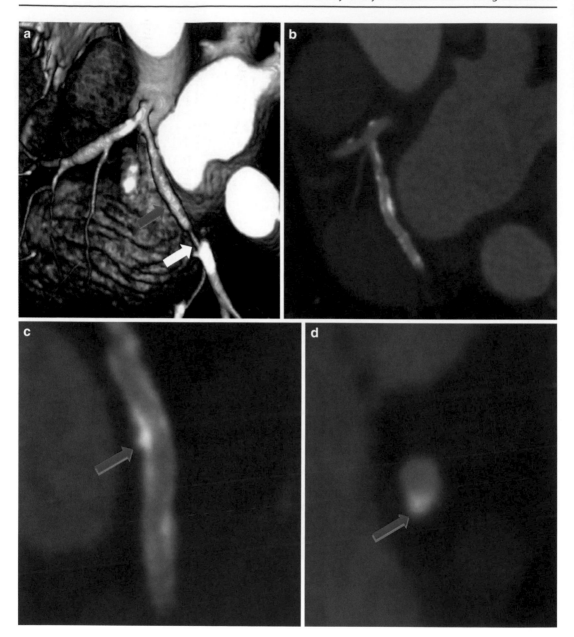

Fig. 4.49 (a) 3D volume rendered image demonstrate stented segment LCX (*blue arrow*) compare it to the non-stented segment (*white arrow*), (b) multiplanar reformat image demonstrate patent stent in mid LCX. (c, d) Multiplanar reformat longitudinal and cross sectional image of the stent demonstrate luminal patency with surrounding calcified plaque (*arrow*)

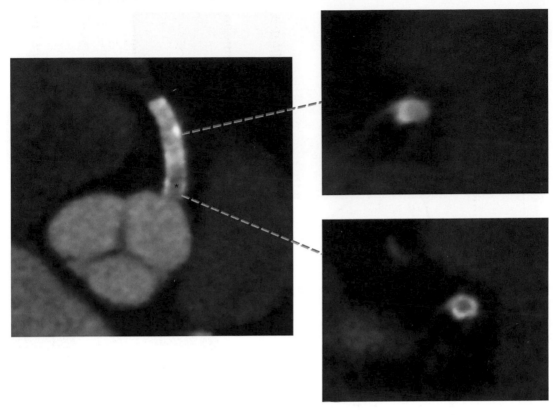

Fig. 4.50 Multiplanar reformat image demonstrate in-stent restenosis in the proximal segment of RCA stent (*), compare the difference in contrast opacification to the completely patent distal segment of the stent on cross sectional images

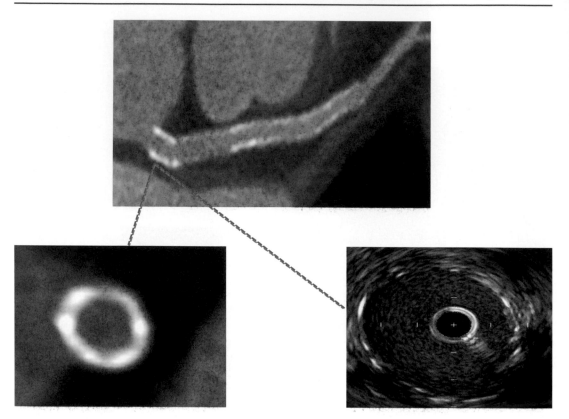

Fig. 4.51 Multiplanar reformat longitudinal and cross sectional image demonstrating patent stent in the left main with IVUS (Intra Vascular Ultra Sound) correlation. Also noted is patent stent in LAD

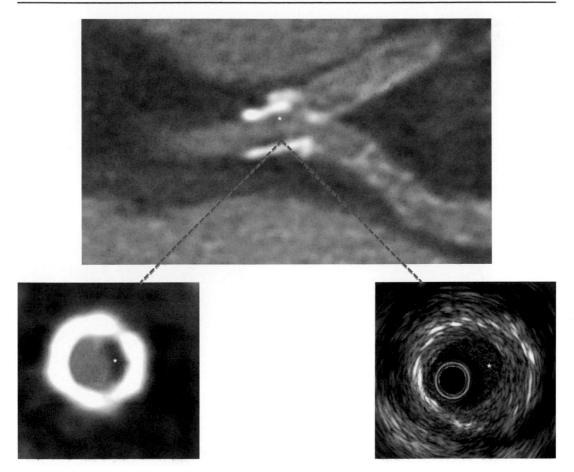

Fig. 4.52 Multiplanar reformat longitudinal and cross sectional image demonstrating left main stent with in stent restenosis (*) with IVUS correlation

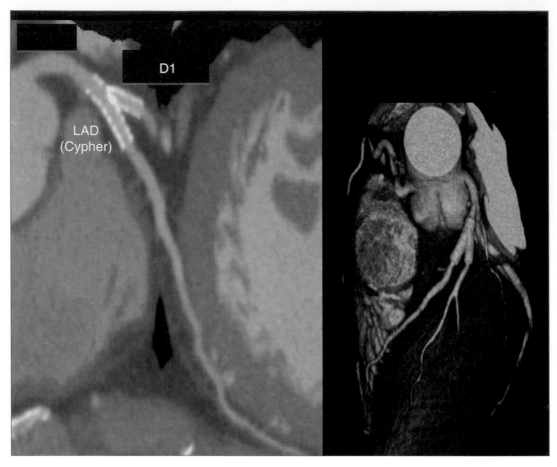

Fig. 4.53 Curved Multiplanar reformat and 3D volume rendered image demonstrate "kissing stents" in proximal LAD and 1st Diagonal branch

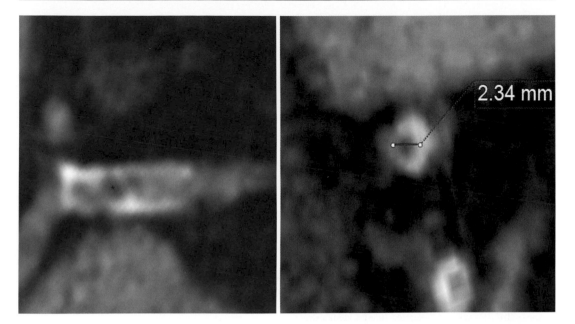

Fig. 4.54 Multiplanar reformat images demonstrate stent in distal LAD. Due to beam hardening artifact accurate assessment of stents become increasingly difficult with diameter <3 mm. In this case it is uncertain whether poor contrast opacification (*) is secondary to beam hardening artifact or in stent restenosis

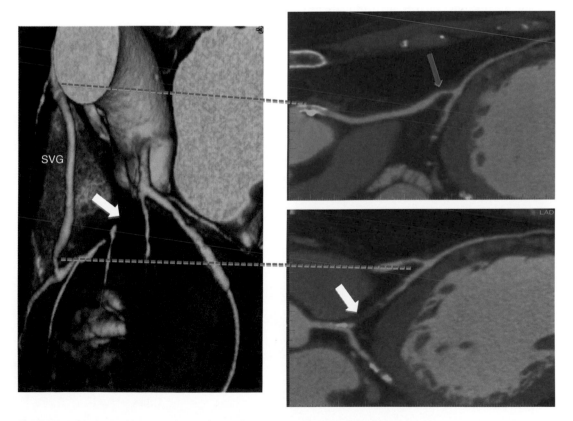

Fig. 4.55 3D volume rendered image demonstrate totally occluded proximal LAD (*white arrow*) with an saphenous vein graft (*SVG*) to mid LAD. Curved multiplanar refor- mat images above demonstrate a stent in proximal seg- ment of vein graft, while the distal segment has obstructive noncalcified plaque (*blue arrow*)

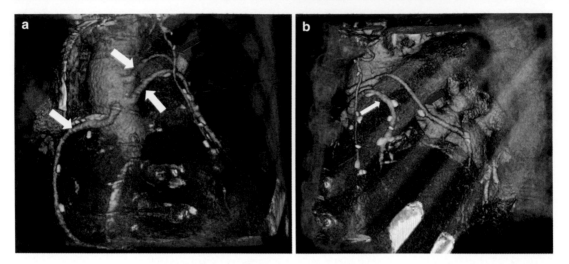

Fig. 4.56 (**a**) 3D volume rendered image in anteroposterior veiw demonstrate three Saphenous vein grafts (*white arrows*) and a Left internal mammary artery graft (*Blue arrow*). (**b**) 3D volume rendered image demonstrate saphenous vein grafts to diagonal branch (*white arrow*), obtuse marginal branch (*blue arrow*) and a Left internal mammary artery graft to mid LAD (*black arrow*)

Note
3D volume rendered images are extremely helpful to begin with when dealing with a bypass graft case. You can assess the number and patency of grafts

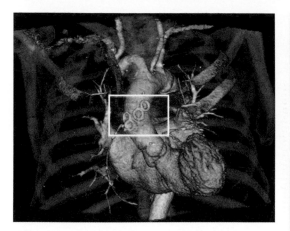

Fig. 4.57 3D volume rendered image demonstrate surgical rings at the vein graft aortic anastomosis, these serves as markers during coronary angiography

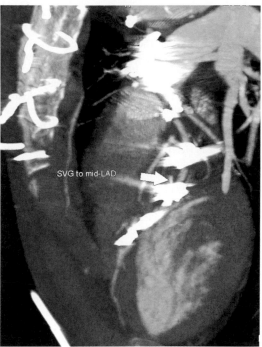

Fig. 4.59 Maximum Intensity projection image demonstrate saphenous vein to mid LAD graft (*white arrow*), extensive blooming artifact results in nondiagnostic image quality

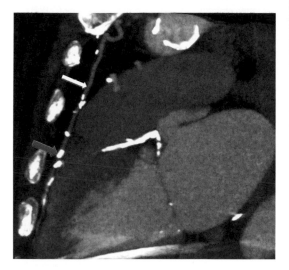

Fig. 4.58 Maximum intensity projection image demonstrate a LIMA graft to distal LAD (*white arrow*). Blooming artifact from surgical clips (To close off side branches) obscure the lumen (*blue arrow*)

References

1. Margolis JR, et al. The diagnostic and prognostic significance of coronary artery calcification. A report of 800 cases. Radiology. 1980;137(3):609–16.
2. Kondos GT, et al. Electron-beam tomography coronary artery calcium and cardiac events: a 37-month follow-up of 5635 initially asymptomatic low- to intermediate-risk adults. Circulation. 2003;107(20):2571–6.
3. O'Rourke RA, et al. American College of Cardiology/American Heart Association Expert Consensus document on electron-beam computed tomography for the diagnosis and prognosis of coronary artery disease. Circulation. 2000;102(1):126–40.
4. Budoff MJ, et al. Long-term prognosis associated with coronary calcification: observations from a registry of 25,253 patients. J Am Coll Cardiol. 2007; 49(18):1860–70.
5. Detrano R, et al. Coronary calcium as a predictor of coronary events in four racial or ethnic groups. N Engl J Med. 2008;358(13):1336–45.
6. Polonsky TS, et al. Coronary artery calcium score and risk classification for coronary heart disease prediction. JAMA. 2010;303(16):1610–6.
7. Arad Y, et al. Treatment of asymptomatic adults with elevated coronary calcium scores with atorvastatin, vitamin C, and vitamin E: the St. Francis Heart Study randomized clinical trial. J Am Coll Cardiol. 2005; 46(1):166–72.
8. Kroft LJ, de Roos A, Geleijns J. Artifacts in ECG-synchronized MDCT coronary angiography. AJR Am J Roentgenol. 2007;189(3):581–91.
9. Budoff MJ, et al. Diagnostic performance of 64-multidetector row coronary computed tomographic angiography for evaluation of coronary artery stenosis in individuals without known coronary artery disease: results from the prospective multicenter ACCURACY (Assessment by Coronary Computed Tomographic Angiography of Individuals Undergoing Invasive Coronary Angiography) trial. J Am Coll Cardiol. 2008;52(21):1724–32.
10. Voros S, et al. Coronary atherosclerosis imaging by coronary CT angiography: current status, correlation with intravascular interrogation and meta-analysis. JACC Cardiovasc Imaging. 2011;4(5):537–48.
11. Ehara S, et al. Spotty calcification typifies the culprit plaque in patients with acute myocardial infarction: an intravascular ultrasound study. Circulation. 2004 ;110(22):3424–9.
12. Virmani R, et al. Lessons from sudden coronary death: a comprehensive morphological classification scheme for atherosclerotic lesions. Arterioscler Thromb Vasc Biol. 2000;20(5):1262–75.
13. Glagov S, et al. Compensatory enlargement of human atherosclerotic coronary arteries. N Engl J Med. 1987;316(22):1371–5.
14. Motoyama S, et al. Computed tomographic angiography characteristics of atherosclerotic plaques subsequently resulting in acute coronary syndrome. J Am Coll Cardiol. 2009;54(1):49–57.
15. Raff GL, et al. Diagnostic accuracy of noninvasive coronary angiography using 64-slice spiral computed tomography. J Am Coll Cardiol. 2005;46(3):552–7.
16. Raff GL, et al. SCCT guidelines for the interpretation and reporting of coronary computed tomographic angiography. J Cardiovasc Comput Tomogr. 2009;3(2):122–36.
17. Rispler S, et al. Integrated single-photon emission computed tomography and computed tomography coronary angiography for the assessment of hemodynamically significant coronary artery lesions. J Am Coll Cardiol. 2007;49(10):1059–67.
18. George RT, et al. Diagnostic performance of combined noninvasive coronary angiography and myocardial perfusion imaging using 320-MDCT: the CT angiography and perfusion methods of the CORE320 multicenter multinational diagnostic study. AJR Am J Roentgenol. 2011;197(4):829–37.
19. Achenbach S, et al. Detection of calcified and noncalcified coronary atherosclerotic plaque by contrast-enhanced, submillimeter multidetector spiral computed tomography: a segment-based comparison with intravascular ultrasound. Circulation. 2004;109(1):14–7.
20. Schoenhagen P, et al. Non-invasive assessment of plaque morphology and remodeling in mildly stenotic coronary segments: comparison of 16-slice computed tomography and intravascular ultrasound. Coron Artery Dis. 2003;14(6):459–62.
21. Hoffmann U, et al. Noninvasive assessment of plaque morphology and composition in culprit and stable lesions in acute coronary syndrome and stable lesions in stable angina by multidetector computed tomography. J Am Coll Cardiol. 2006;47(8):1655–62.
22. Schmermund A, Mohlenkamp S, Schlosser T, Raimund E. Coronary angiography after revascularization. In: Budoff MJ, Shinbane JS, editors. Cardiac CT imaging: diagnosis of cardiovascular disease. London: Springer; 2006. p. 135–45.
23. Jen-Sho Chen J, White C. CT angiography for coronary artery bypass graft surgery. Appl Radiol. 2008;37:10–8.
24. Martuscelli E. Coronary artery bypass grafts. In: Dewey M, editor. Cardiac CT. Berlin: Springer; 2011. p. 171–8.
25. Anders K. Coronary artery stents. In: Dewey M, editor. Cardiac CT. Berlin: Springer; 2011. p. 179–90.
26. Mahnken A. CT imaging of coronary stents: past, present, and future. ISRN Cardiol. 2012;2012:1–12.

Utilization of CCTA for Structural Diseases

5

Ammar Chaudhry and Muzammil H. Musani

The objective of this chapter is to outline basic epidemiology, pathophysiology, clinical presentation, and imaging findings of common structural heart disease. Structural heart disease can result from a variety of processes effecting the myocardium, pericardium, vasculature, or cardiac valves. This chapter will outline disease processes effecting the aforementioned and highlight imaging findings that can aid in diagnosis and patient management.

5.1 Myocardial Infarction

Myocardial infarction (MI) results from the occlusion of coronary arteries most commonly from atherosclerotic plaque rupture followed by thrombosis leading to ischemia and myocyte damage [1–5]. Patients generally present with chest pain which may radiate to the jaw or arm, dyspnea, hemodynamic instability, etc. [1–5]. Patient evaluation varies within regions and hospitals, generally depending on the expertise available within the institution. In most cases, initial evaluation generally involves obtaining an electrocardiogram and cardiac enzymes [2]. Mortality in acute MI is approximately 20 % with 6 % in hospital mortality [1–3]. Given this, urgent revascularization is stressed in setting of acute MI. Patients with positive initial findings (elevated cardiac enzymes, ECG changes, etc.) are taken for interventional or surgical revascularization. If the aforementioned are unremarkable for

ST-elevation MI (STEMI), patients may be observed with serial cardiac enzymes, get stress myocardial perfusion exam, or get a CCTA [1, 2]. In such cases, ECG-gated CCTA evaluation can demonstrate the degree of vessel occlusion (coronary artery filling defect with or without adjacent calcific plaque), myocardial hypoattenuation, and wall-motion abnormalities (hypokinetic, akinetic, or dyskinetic) in acute setting. CCTA can also detect presence of valvular dysfunction, septal or papillary muscle rupture in massive MI [1–3]. Secondary signs of an MI including pericarditis, pericardial effusion, CHF (pulmonary vascular congestion, pleural effusions, etc.) can also be detected. In chronic stages, myocardial thinning, aneurysmal changes, and dystrophic calcifications can be seen [2–4]. Echocardiogram can show wall-motion abnormalities, septal and papillary muscle involvement, and presence of pericardial effusion, however, not to the degree of anatomic detail seen on CCTA. Additionally, the degree of vessel occlusion and extracardiac findings are not seen on echocardiography. MRI can demonstrate findings seen on CCTA. One of the key benefits of MRI is that it provides a precise assessment of myocardial stunning and identifying viable myocardium, which aids in determining interventional management (CABG versus stenting) [6, 7]. Additionally, MRI is the most accurate means of assessing cardiac output and the extent of myocardial involvement [6, 7]. One important limitation of MRI at present is motion artifact (cardiac and respiratory) which can limit evaluation of coronary arteries. These limitations limit the utility of MRI in an acute setting, as accurate knowledge of degree of coronary artery occlusion is the base of patient management. Therefore, at present, MRI is generally used in subacute and chronic settings [2–4, 6, 7].

5.2   Left Atrial and Left Atrial Appendage Thrombus

Thrombus formation in the left atrial body (LAB) and/or the left atrial appendage (LAA) is generally seen in setting of atrial fibrillation or mitral valve stenosis [8–10]. These conditions result in slow blood flow in the LAB and LAA which leads to formation of a thrombus. The thrombus, especially if mobile, is at increased risk of embolization [8, 10–13]. Echocardiography is generally the initial imaging modality used, and it can reveal an echogenic clot in the body of the left atrium or in the left atrial appendage [11–13]. Chronic thrombus (especially if broad based) can develop neovascularity which can lead to presence of Doppler signal, thus can mimic an atrial neoplasm [11–13]. Thrombus on ECG-gated CCTA appears as a hypoattenuated filling defect in LAB and/or LAA. If there is heterogeneity in IV contrast distribution especially in the LAA, then a one-minute delayed CCTA scan can be obtained. Persistence of LAB/LAA filling defect is highly suggestive of a thrombus. If LAA is completely contrast opacified, then the filling defect seen on initial images is likely slow-flow artifact. MRI can also detect LAB/LAA thrombus [8, 11–13]. There are variable appearance of the clot on T1 and T2 sequences depending on the level of hemoglobin (oxygenated, deoxygenated) and hemosiderin present. LAA/LAB thrombus on postcontrast MRI will appear as a filling defect that persists on delayed images [10–13]. Anticoagulation reduces the risk of embolic events [10–13].

5.3   Dilated Cardiomyopathy

Dilated cardiomyopathy (DCM) refers to enlargement of cardiac chambers and contractile dysfunction resulting in heart failure (ejection fraction

<40 %) [14, 15]. It usually is biventricular and can be subacute to chronic, resulting from a multitude of causes. The most common cause is ischemic cardiomyopathy in the US and is most prevalent in the elderly usually with risk factors of coronary artery disease [14, 15]. Overall prognosis depends on degree of left ventricular dysfunction [14, 15, 18]. Additionally, older age, male gender, and race (African American) statistically have worse prognosis. Subacute and chronic causes of DCM include myocarditis (infectious, autoimmune conditions), peripartum cardiomyopathy, and drug toxicity (chemotherapy agents, cocaine), metabolic (hypophosphatemia, uremia, hypocalcemia), and endocrinopathies (thyroid dysfunction, Cushing disease, etc.) [14–18]. Idiopathic DCM is the most common cause worldwide and familial DCM accounts for 25 % of these cases [19, 20]. Differential considerations for DCM include restrictive cardiomyopathy, hypertrophic cardiomyopathy, and valvular heart disease [14–18]. Patients usually present with signs and symptoms of heart failure (gradual development of dyspnea on exertion, orthopnea, paroxysmal nocturnal dyspnea, peripheral edema, etc.) [14, 15].

On chest radiographs, the diagnosis can be suggested by widened cardiac silhouette occupying greater than 50 % of the thorax width on posterior-anterior (PA) view. Secondary signs of heart failure can be seen including pulmonary vascular congestion, dilated azygous vein, and pleural effusions [14–17]. Usually if there are signs and symptoms of dilated cardiomyopathies, transthoracic echocardiography (TEE) is the most common initial modality used to evaluate dilated cardiomyopathy. TTE can reveal wall-motion abnormalities, valvular dysfunction, and cardiac chamber volumes; however, given the lack of specificity and variability in ejection fraction, additional modalities are used to evaluate DCM [14, 15, 17].

Cardiac CTA (CCTA) can be used to rule out the most common cause of DCM, i.e., ischemia with high degree of sensitivity and specificity. Ventricular dimensions and volume can be obtained accurately. Newer volume rendered multiphase techniques can help obtain estimated ejection fractions. CCTA is useful in acute setting as the scan can be performed quickly and yields fairly accurate results. Additionally, newer techniques are allowing for assessment of myocardial perfusion with accuracy comparable to those seen in MRI and cardiac nuclear medicine tests [22, 23].

Magnetic resonance imaging (MRI) is the most accurate method for assessing dilated cardiomyopathy as it can give accurate assessment of cardiac chamber size and ventricular ejection fractions [14, 15, 21]. Ventricular dimensions, volume, and ejection fractions can be obtained accurately. In addition, detailed cardiac anatomy can be obtained [21]. However, MRI is limited in evaluating coronary arteries, limiting its utility in acute setting. Thus, CCTA is the preferred modality in evaluating patients in acute to subacute settings to exclude ischemic cardiomyopathy, and MRI can be used for problem solving in equivocal cases.

Treatment usually entails addressing reversible cause such as revascularization in cases of ischemic DCM, steroids (autoimmune), and cardiac transplant. In addition, symptoms are treated with medical therapy (ACE inhibitors, beta-blockers, diuretics, and antiarrhythmic agents) [14, 15, 18].

5.4   Left Ventricular Aneurysm

Left ventricular aneurysm (LVA) refers to a thin fibrotic segment of left ventricular myocardium which may be dyskinetic or akinetic [24, 25]. It most commonly results from prior transmural myocardial infarction and is most commonly seen in anterior and apical segments secondary to left anterior descending artery occlusion [26]. Infrequently, inferior-basal wall aneurysms may be seen after right coronary artery territory transmural infarcts [26]. It develops in approximately eight-to-fifteen percent of patients with ST-elevation myocardial infarction (STEMI) [24–26]. Most LVAs are asymptomatic but can lead to systolic dysfunction [24–26]. Large-sized LVA can have slow blood flow that can lead to the formation of thrombus which can subsequently embolize [24–26]. Additionally, LVA can serve as foci of arrhythmias that can be fatal. Overall, patients with STEMI and resultant LVA have worse outcomes than those without LVA [24–26].

LVA can be seen on echocardiography, CCTA, and MRI. Unenhanced cardiac CT can reveal aneurysmal remodeling of the left ventricle with or without calcification in the infarcted myocardium and/or mural thrombus [27, 28]. CCTA reveals thin fibrotic myocardium with wall-motion abnormalities. Occasionally, filling defect can be seen, which represents thrombus in the LVA [27, 28]. The aforementioned findings can be seen on MRI and echocardiography. In addition, MRI can reveal transmural delayed hyperenhancement in the scarred myocardium of the LVA [24, 28, 29]. Treatment generally involves medical management of modifiable cardiovascular risk factors and revascularization in cases where there is viable myocardium present. Antiarrhythmics are used in setting of ventricular arrhythmias, and implantable cardiac defibrillators are used in patients with high risk of sudden cardiac death [24, 26, 29].

5.5   Left Ventricular Thrombus

Left ventricular thrombus (LVT) is generally seen in patients with transmural myocardial infarction with flow disturbance resulting from wall-motion abnormality and/or LV aneurysm [30–33]. Rarely, it can be secondary to tumor thrombus, Takotsubo cardiomyopathy, and chemotherapy [30, 31]. The thrombus can persist and overtime may develop dystrophic calcification. There is increased risk of embolization if the thrombus is large and mobile.

LVT can be seen on echocardiography as an echogenic mass which may be mobile, pedunculated, or adherent to myocardial wall [33–35]. On CCTA, LVT presents as a filling defect in the left ventricle that persists on delayed imaging. Associated wall-motion abnormalities and coronary artery disease can also be seen [32–34]. Chronic thrombus may contain calcifications, which present as hyperdense foci within the aneurysm. On noncontrast images, the thrombus appears slightly lower in attenuation as compared to normal myocardium [32–34]. Thrombus generally appears hyperintense in acute-to-subacute stages on spin-echo sequences and gradually becomes hypointense in chronic stages [30, 31, 33, 36]. Important to note that there can be reactive thrombus that may form around intraventricular mass. There is no postcontrast enhancement seen in a fresh thrombus [30, 31, 33, 36]. Chronic broad-based thrombus may demonstrate minimal postcontrast enhancement due to neovascularity [30, 31, 33, 36]. In such cases, a biopsy may be performed to exclude intracardiac neoplasm. Treatment generally involves rate and rhythm control plus anticoagulation to reduce risk of embolization [36].

5.6   Hypertrophic Obstructive Cardiomyopathy (HOCM)

Hypertrophic obstructive cardiomyopathy (HOCM) is a primary myocardial disorder affecting the sarcomeres resulting in hypertrophy of the left ventricle (LV) [37, 38, 46]. Additional reversible causes of LV hypertrophy should be ruled out including hypertension or aortic valve stenosis [37, 38]. Clinically, patients can be asymptomatic or present with arrhythmias, sudden cardiac arrest (from ventricular fibrillation or sustained ventricular tachycardia), chest pain, and/or signs of decreased cardiac output (e.g., syncope, orthopnea, paroxysmal nocturnal dyspnea) [37, 38]. It is the leading cause of sudden cardiac arrest in young, otherwise healthy, individuals including athletes [37, 38]. Diagnostic criteria include asymmetric LV thickness of greater than 15 mm; however, functional obstruction has been reported where LV thickness was less than 15 mm [37, 39–42]. Ratio of asymmetric septal hypertrophy can also be used to aid in diagnosis and is defined by the ratio of the septal wall thickness to a nonhypertrophied segment greater than 1.3 [39–42]. The most common location is the basal septum which may or may not result in LV outflow obstruction. Additional areas of involvement include the LV mid-cavity and/or apex [37, 39–42]. Classic cases of HOCM are autosomal dominant with incomplete penetrance and variable expressivity resulting in a wide spectrum of clinical and imaging spectrum [38, 46]. Histopathologic evaluation reveals hypertrophied myocytes arranged in disorganized bundles surrounded by expanded interstitial compartment containing variable degree of collagen deposition (fibrosis) [38].

Echocardiography, generally first diagnostic imaging modality to be used, can show nondilated and/or hyperdynamic left ventricle with variable degree of hypertrophic changes which can result in left ventricular outflow tract obstruction [43]. In severe cases of HOCM, mitral valve regurgitation and/or systolic anterior motion of the mitral valve leaflet can be seen [37, 43]. CCTA and MR imaging can show all the echocardiography finding more precisely and yield more reliable/reproducible measurements [40]. Additionally, MRI can reveal areas of increased fibrosis (delayed hyperenhancement on postcontrast images) which can serve as arrhythmogenic foci and the total volume of delayed hyperenhancement on MRI correlates with risk for sudden cardiac arrest [37, 39–44]. Treatment generally revolves around optimizing cardiac function, which can be done by using beta-blockers and calcium channel blockers to improve diastolic relaxation which results in improved ventricular filling and also reduces risk of arrhythmias. Interventional therapies include permanent pacemaker placement, septal myomectomy, or septal ablation [43, 44]. Automatic implantable defibrillators are used in patients with high risk for sudden cardiac death [43, 44].

5.7   Myocardial Bridging

Myocardial bridging refers to congenital variance in the course of coronary artery which instead of taking its normal epicardial course, takes an intramyocardial course [45, 46]. The degree of bridging is variable generally involving a small segment of the vessel and most patients are asymptomatic [45, 46]. Symptoms, when they occur, are generally during time of maximal systole; myocardial contraction constricts intramyocardial segment of the coronary artery resulting in ischemia and rarely infarction [45]. Severity of symptoms varies depending on the coronary artery involved and the degree of resultant stenosis. Most patients have isolated myocardial bridging; however, in some instances, multiple segments and/or multiple vessels can be involved [45, 46]. The most common location is the mid left anterior descending artery (LAD), followed by left circumflex artery (LCx), and right coronary artery (RCA) [45, 46]. Increased sheer stress in arterial segment proximal to the myocardial bridge predisposes to atherosclerosis [45, 46]. Interestingly, a higher incidence is noted in patients with hypertrophic cardiomyopathy, for reasons poorly understood. Complications include vasospasm, ventricular septal rupture, arrhythmias, myocardial stunning, and sudden cardiac arrest [45, 47].

Coronary computed tomographic angiography (CCTA) is the best imaging modality which depicts intramyocardial locations of coronary artery [45–47]. Echocardiography has limited role in diagnosis of myocardial bridging. MRI can show myocardial imaging; however, motion artifact limits detection of small segment lesions [45–47]. Treatment generally involves rhythm and rate control and in certain cases interventions including percutaneous coronary artery stenting and coronary artery bypass can be performed [45–47].

5.8   Fatty Infiltration of RV (ARVC)

Fatty infiltration of right ventricle, also referred to as arrhythmogenic right ventricular cardiomyopathy (ARVC), is typified by fibrofatty degeneration of the right ventricle which can lead to dysrhythmias and potentially sudden cardiac death [48–51]. It generally presents with syncope, ventricular arrhythmias, and sudden cardiac death [48–51]. Histopathologic evaluation reveals fibrofatty infiltration of the right ventricular myocardium, most commonly involving the anterior wall. ARVC can have a patchy involvement of the myocardium, thus, can result in false negative biopsy. Diagnosis is confirmed with presence of greater than 3 % fibrous tissue and greater than 49 % fat, with the process beginning in the subepicardium and extending endocardially. Autopsy studies have demonstrated involvement of left ventricle as well (40–76 %) [48–51].

Diagnosis is made using combination of clinical and imaging findings. Diagnosis is suggested

by fulfilling two major criteria, one major and two minor criteria or four minor criteria [48–52]. Major criteria include RV global dilatation and RV aneurysm, which can be seen on various imaging modalities. Family history, if biopsy proven, is considered major criteria. Minor criteria include ECG abnormalities, regional RV wall-motion abnormalities, and family history of ARVD without pathology proven diagnosis is considered minor criteria [48–52].

Various imaging modalities can aid in diagnosing ARVC, including echocardiography, coronary computed tomographic angiography (CCTA), and magnetic resonance imaging (MRI) [48–51]. Diagnosis of ARVC on imaging is suggested by dilated right ventricle, right ventricular aneurysm, and/or thickened trabeculae. CCTA can reveal dilated right ventricle, reduced systolic function, and RV aneurysm [48–51]. CCTA can also demonstrate intramyocardial macroscopic fat; however, sensitivity and specificity of this is not well established and is under clinical investigation [48–51]. MRI can demonstrate variable degree of fatty infiltration of the myocardium, which is considered major criteria. The extent of myocardial involvement can be appreciated on T1 pre- and post-contrast fat suppressed sequences where the myocardial fat is suppressed by the MR pulse signal thus appearing as hypointense focus within the myocardium [48–51]. The degree of myocardial fibrosis is variable and can have a patchy distribution. These changes can be seen on MRI as areas of delayed hyperenhancement. Wall-motion abnormalities can be appreciated on MRI and echocardiography [48–51]. Treatment usually involves avoiding rigorous exercise or activities that would result in increased sympathetic tone of the heart. Beta-blockers are used in the absence of arrhythmias and/or implantable cardioverter defibrillator. Antiarrhythmics are used in cases with dysrhythmias [52].

5.9   Noncompacted Cardiomyopathy

Noncompacted cardiomyopathy (NCM) is associated with several deep trabeculations of ventricular wall that communicate with ventricular chamber resulting in abnormal ventricular motion and diminished cardiac output [53, 54]. It most commonly involves the left ventricle and referred to as left ventricular noncompaction (LVNC) [53, 54]. Patients generally present with signs and symptoms of heart failure including dyspnea, orthopnea, hemodynamic instability, etc. [55]. Tachyarrhythmias and embolic complications can be seen [55]. LVNC can be an isolated finding or be seen with congenital heart disease. Prognostic indicators include number of effected segments, diastolic dysfunction, and heart failure at presentation [53–55].

On echocardiography, CCTA, and MRI, there is visualization of distinct two-layered appearance of trabeculated (noncompacted) myocardium and compact myocardium generally involving the left ventricular apex and/or mid and distal segments of inferior and lateral walls [53–56]. Echocardiography is generally the first modality used. CCTA and/or MRI is used to gain more precise anatomic and functional information, which is especially helpful in surgical planning [53–56]. Treatment revolves around management of heart failure, tachyarrhythmia, and/or embolic disease [53–56].

5.10   Infectious Endocarditis

Infectious endocarditis, as the name implies, involves infection of the heart most commonly the valves with infrequent involvement of the cardiac chambers [57–60]. Common infectious agents include *Staphylococcus* and *Streptococcus* species and rarely can be secondary to tuberculosis, fungal organisms, and form HACEK organisms (*Hemophilus, Actinobacillus, Cardiobacterium, Eikenella, Kingella*) [57–60]. Diagnosis is made on combination of clinical, laboratory, and imaging findings using modified Duke Criteria (major and minor). Major criteria include positive blood cultures and positive echocardiography findings (vegetation, new regurgitant valve). Minor criteria include fever (>38 °C), risk factors (IV-drug abuse or predisposing cardiac conditions, e.g., valvular disease, prosthetic valve, pacemaker),

vascular involvement (arterial embolic to lung, brain, liver, kidney, etc.), and immunological findings (e.g., osler nodes, positive rheumatoid factor). Need to fulfill two major or one major and three minor criteria to confirm diagnosis of endocarditis [57–59, 62]. Note, however, given early treatment and delayed complications, the modified Duke criteria may not be present on initial presentation [57–59, 62]. Complications including septic emboli, valvular cusp perforation, perivalvular abscess, pseudoaneurysm, and/or fistula portend poor prognosis with reported mortality up to 40 % [57–59, 62]. Risk of embolic disease is increased in patients with mobile vegetations and/or vegetation size greater than 1 cm [57–59, 62].

Initial imaging modality is usually transthoracic echocardiography (TEE) which may demonstrate vegetations, which appear as oscillating irregular-shaped mass adherent to the valve and/or endocardium [57–59, 62, 66, 67]. Complications including regurgitation, abscess, and pseudoaneurysm may be seen on TEE. However, due to the poor sensitivity and specificity of TEE, transthoracic echocardiography is used which yields modest improvement in sensitivity and specificity. However, given TEE's invasive nature and use of anesthesia, alternative diagnostic modalities can be used especially in more critically ill patients whose clinical course may get complicated with an invasive procedure and/or patients who may not tolerate anesthesia/intubation [57–59, 62, 66, 67]. ECG-gated cardiac computed tomographic angiography (CCTA) can detect valvular vegetations, perivalvular or aortic root abscess, and pseudoaneurysm with a similar sensitivity and specificity as compared to TEE [60–67]. Pseudoaneurysm presents as contrast filled space in communication with the cardiac chamber and/or aortic root. Leaflet perforation, though difficult to detect, presents as discontinuity in a cusp [61–67]. Fistula can vary in size and is represented by communication between cardiac chambers [61–67]. The benefits of CCTA is that it is noninvasive, rapidly performed, provides better anatomic detail, which can aid in surgical planning, if needed. Additionally, CCTA can provide information on involvement of the coronary arteries and septic pulmonary emboli. MRI can reveal cardiac involvement of infectious endocarditis with slightly improved sensitivity and specificity; however, given the critical state of the patients and long duration of the MRI exam, CCTA should be considered [61–67]. Also, CCTA is the preferred modality to detect pulmonary involvement. Treatment involves long-term intravenous antibiotic. Surgical treatment may be required in complications including large vegetations, severe valvular regurgitation, pseudoaneurysm, abscess, and fistulae [57–59, 65, 67].

5.11 Aortic Root Abscess

Aortic root abscess is not an uncommon complication of infectious endocarditis and is seen in approximately 30–40 % [67–69]. Patients usually present with persistent bacteremia and develop new conduction defects in spite of appropriate course of antibiotics [67, 69, 70]. Aortic valve and aortic annulus are more prone to abscess formation for reasons unclear and the abscess can further extend into adjacent myocardium (especially when involves the right and noncoronary cusps), destroying conductive tissue resulting in heart block [68–70]. The aortic root abscess can also rarely extend up to and occlude the coronary arteries resulting in myocardial ischemia/infarction [70]. In infectious endocarditis, aortic root/perivalvular abscess portends poor prognosis with mortality rates twice as high rates of mortality, usually secondary to systemic embolization [67, 68].

Transthoracic echocardiography (TEE), despite its low sensitive (28 %) is usually the first study used to evaluate potential aortic root abscess [67, 69, 71]. Transesophageal echocardiography (TEE) is the second modality used with sensitivity and specificity of 87 and 95 %, respectively [67, 69, 71]. Although TEE is more sensitive, it still can miss more than one in ten patients with aortic root abscess [67, 69, 71].

ECG-gated coronary computed tomographic angiography (CCTA) can be used to evaluate aortic root abscess with high sensitivity and specificity [72]. The noninvasive nature of the technique,

with great anatomic detail, makes it a viable option for evaluating patients with suspicion of aortic root abscess, especially those who are too sick to undergo general anesthesia required for TEE [72]. In addition to localization of the abscess, CCTA can evaluate extent of the abscess and exclude involvement of coronary arteries, which the TEE/TTE is unable to do [72].

5.12 Pericardial Effusion, Pericardial Calcification, and Constrictive Pericarditis

Pericardial calcifications can result from prior trauma, pericarditis (infectious, autoimmune, uremic, radiation, etc.), postsurgical, or be idiopathic [73–80]. The distribution or appearance of pericardial calcification is nonspecific, and diagnosis is generally made based on clinical findings [73–77, 80]. Constrictive pericarditis is a key diagnosis one must exclude when evaluating patients with pericardial calcifications as it can result in hemodynamic changes, chest pain, and congestive heart failure [80]. Echocardiography is used as primary imaging modality due to its cost, availability, and portability [77, 80]. Characteristic findings of constrictive pericarditis on echocardiography include early diastolic filling with rapid with elevation and equalization of intrachamber diastolic pressures [77, 80]. Abnormal septal motion and absent inspiratory collapse of IVC are secondary signs suggestive of constrictive pericarditis [77, 80]. Given limitations and decreased sensitivity and specificity of TTE and limited scanned field of view of TEE, echocardiograph is limited in assessment of constrictive pericarditis. CT and MRI provide a more complete evaluation [73–80]. On CCTA, combination of pericardial thickening (greater than 4–6 mm), pericardial enhancement, plus peri-/epicardial fat stranding raise the possibility of pericarditis [75, 76]. Impaired ventricular filling (presence of dilated superior and inferior vena cava along with tubular ventricles) is suggestive of constrictive physiology [75, 76]. The presence of calcifications further support the diagnosis of constrictive pericarditis, especially if greater than fifty percent of pericardium is calcified [75, 76]. Pericardial calcifications are best seen on CCTA as hyperdense foci which may be linear or nodular and may be segmental or circumferential in distribution [75, 76]. CCTA can also demonstrate extracardiac manifestations of constrictive pericarditis, including pulmonary vascular congestion, pleural and pericardial effusions, hepatic venous congestion, ascites, etc. [73–80]. CT can help characterize pericardial effusion. Hemopericardium on unenhanced images appear as hyperdense fluid measuring 40–60 Hounsfield Units. Pericardial effusion measuring less than 20 Hounsfield units is likely simple and transudative. Pericardial effusion ranging from 20 to 40 Hounsfield units is indeterminate, can be transudative or exudative, and requires clinical correlation [75, 76]. MRI can demonstrate the aforementioned with variable degree of sensitivity and specificity. MRI is more sensitive and specific in characterizing pericardial effusion and detect presence of myocardial involvement as compared to CCTA and echocardiography. MRI and echocardiography are less sensitive techniques for detection of pericardial calcification and are generally not used to evaluate pericardial calcifications [73–77, 79, 80]. Reversible and/or modifiable factors (uremia, inflammation, infections, etc.) are managed medically. Stable, asymptomatic patients without constrictive physiology are generally observed. Severely symptomatic patients or those with constrictive physiology undergo surgical stripping of the pericardium [73–80].

5.13 Pericardial Cyst

Pericardial cyst is a benign congenital mediastinal cyst attached to the pericardium [75, 76]. These cysts can be congenital (resulting from the embryologic defect in the coelomic cavity) or acquired (posttraumatic, sequela of pericarditis) [75, 76, 81–83]. It is usually an incidental finding. Size of the cyst varies from 2 cm up to 30 cm [75, 76, 81–83]. On imaging, it presents as a smoothly marginated fluid collection adjacent to the heart, usually in the right anterior cardiophrenic angle [75, 76, 81–83]. Echocardiography can demonstrate an anechoic mass in the pericardial space. Presence of internal septations help discriminate unilocular from a multilocular cyst [75, 76, 81–83]. On CCTA, the cyst appears as a low attenuation (less than 20 Hounsfield units) smooth homogenous mass with imperceptible walls, without internal enhancement, calcifications, and with or without internal septations [75, 76, 81–83]. MRI is the most sensitive and specific modality; however, cost and image scan time have limited the use of MRI as first line. At present, MRI is generally used for problem solving and to exclude neoplasm [75, 76, 81–84]. For example, MRI is used in cases where the cyst may contain equivocal internal echoes or Doppler flow on ultrasound, equivocal internal, peripheral or septal enhancement of the cyst [84]. Cases where MRI findings are equivocal or nondiagnostic, close follow-up and/or biopsy can be performed to exclude cystic neoplasm [84].

5.14 Pericardial Mass

Pericardial masses may be primary or secondary neoplasms [84, 88, 92, 94]. Secondary neoplasms are more common than primary and result from direct invasion (lymphoma, lung or breast cancer), or from hematogenous or lymphatic spread (melanoma, carcinoid, leukemia) [84, 88, 92, 94]. Rarely, pericardial mass may represent a primary cardiac/pericardiac neoplasm: usually a sarcomatous lesion with angiosarcoma being the most common lesion [95]. Most pericardial masses are asymptomatic and are found incidentally. Symptoms occur due to invasion of adjacent structures (pain if bone invasion), mass effect of the mass on adjacent structures resulting (e.g., cardiac compression resulting in constrictive/restrictive physiology) [94–96].

Imaging aids in diagnosis of pericardial lesions and helps discriminate pericardial masses from pericardial cyst (benign). It also aids in surgical management by providing information on involvement of adjacent structures (involvement of pericardium, myocardium, pleura, lung, bones, etc.), vascular supply, and possible presence of additional lesions [84–96]. Echocardiography demonstrates a pericardial mass with variable echogenicity and Doppler flow [94, 96]. Evaluation on echocardiography is limited due to limited acoustic windows. CCTA and MRI may demonstrate thickened, irregular pericardium with a homogenous to heterogeneous mass with variable degree of enhancement [84–96]. The imaging characteristics depend on tumor grade and histological subtype. Secondary findings including additional lesions (mediastinum, pleura, lungs, and bones), coronary artery involvement, pericardial effusion, constrictive/restrictive physiology, etc., can also be seen. In equivocal cases, positron emission tomography (PET) can be used to evaluate for FDG avidity, which is generally higher in neoplastic processes than benign conditions [94–96]. Treatment and prognosis depends on tumor stage and histologic subtypes. In general, primary cardiac tumors (angiosarcoma) or widespread metastases (melanoma, etc.) have poor prognosis [94–96].

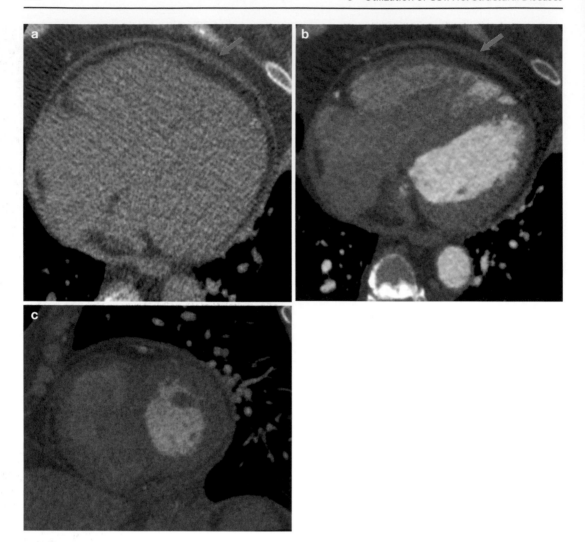

Fig. 5.1 Noncontrast cardiac CT in the axial plane (**a**) reveals diffuse pericardial soft tissue attenuation (*blue arrow*) measuring 5–8 mm anteriorly, without pericardial calcification. *The concentric nature of the soft tissue attenuation is most consistent with diffuse pericardial thickening. A con-* *trast-enhanced MRI may be useful in differentiating between enhancing thickened pericardium and fluid.* Postcontrast arterial phase images in the axial (**b**) and short axis planes (**c**) also demonstrate similar findings (*blue arrow*). *Postcontrast CT is insensitive for pericardial enhancement*

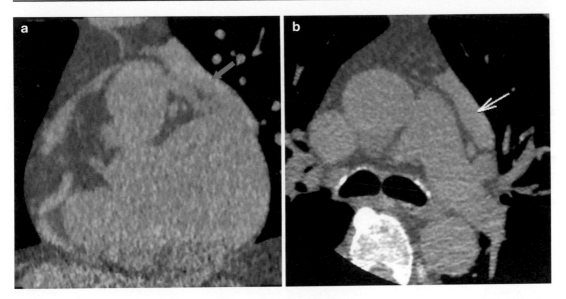

Fig. 5.2 Noncontrast cardiac CT in the straight coronal and axial planes (**a**, **b**) reveals focal soft tissue attenuation (*blue arrow*) along the anterosuperior pericardium (*white arrow*), which may represent focal pericardial thickening versus less likely a loculated pericardial effusion.

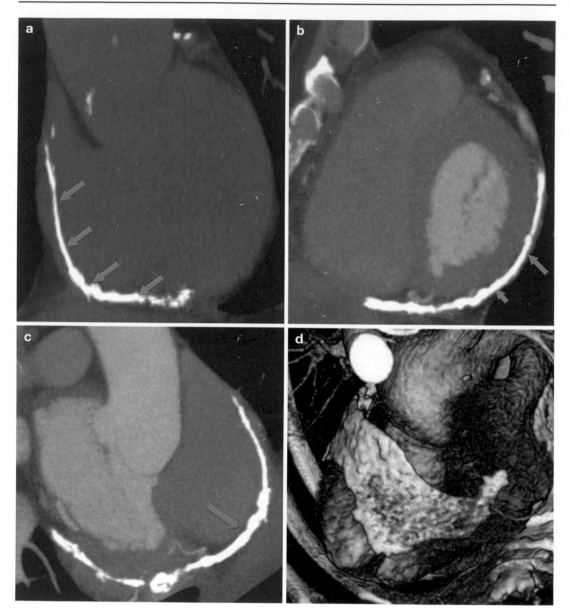

Fig. 5.3 Multiplanar maximum intensity projection (**a–c**) and volume rendered (**d**) images reveal dense sheetlike pericardial calcification (*blue arrows*) enveloping the base of the heart from lateral LV wall to the superior vena cava consistent with sequelae of remote pericarditis

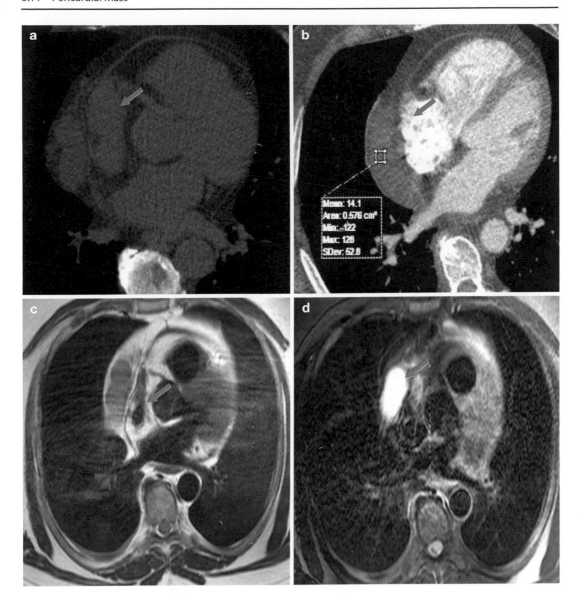

Fig. 5.4 Axial multiplanar reformat noncontrast cardiac CT (**a**) reveals abnormal low density well-circumscribed lesion (*blue arrow*) without evidence of enhancement on postcontrast images (**b**). MRI of the same patient demon-strates T1 hypointense (**c**) and T2 hyperintense (**d**) well-circumscribed lesion (*blue arrow*) without mass effect or mediastinal infiltration, most consistent with a pericardial cyst

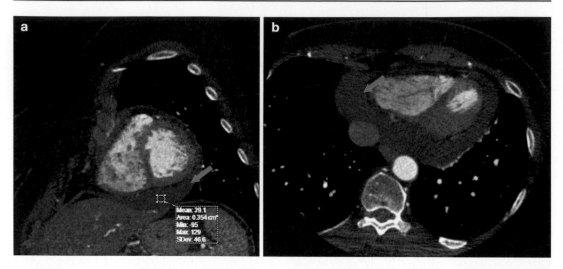

Fig. 5.5 Short axis IV contrast-enhanced CCTA image at the level of the apex demonstrates high attenuating pericardial fluid (HU=39) at the inferior aspect of the heart (*blue arrow*). Axial IV contrast-enhanced CCTA at the inferior aspect of the heart demonstrates a homogenously low attenuation (*blue arrow*) pericardial effusion (**a, b**)

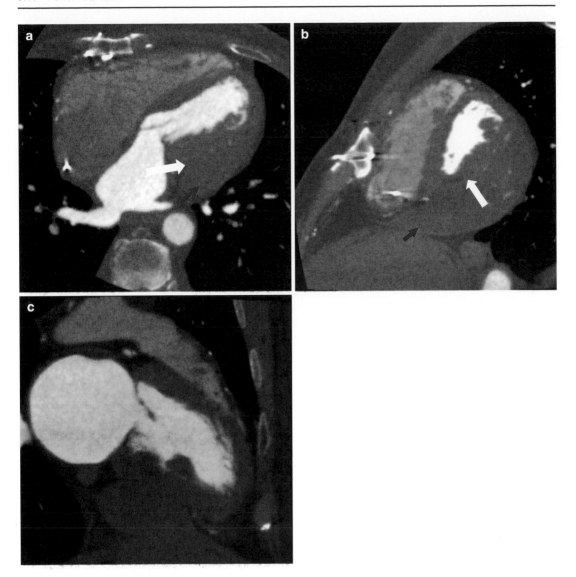

Fig. 5.6 Multiplanar reformats including four-chamber view (**a**); short-axis (**b**); and two-chamber vies (**c**) demonstrate a heterogenously enhancing pericardial mass (*red arrows*) abutting the compressed left ventricle (*white arrows*)

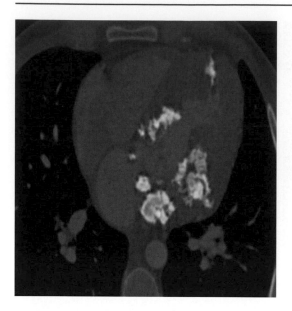

Fig. 5.7 (**a**) Maximum intensity projection in four chamber view demonstrates extensive myocardial calcification of the left ventricle. MRI (not shown) revealed signal drop-off in regions of myocardial calcifications

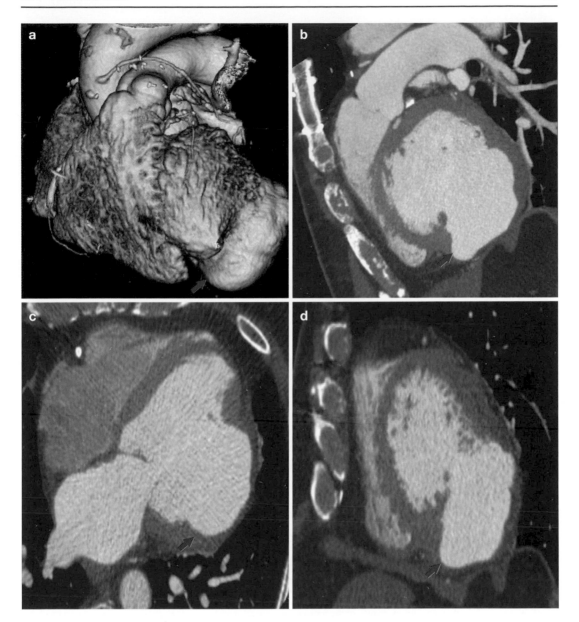

Fig. 5.8 Volume rendered image (**a**) demonstrates abnormal contour and out-pouching of the left ventricle. Maximum intensity projection of the right ventricular outflow tract view (**b**) demonstrates a larger left ventricular pseudoaneurysm. There is no evidence of thrombus in the aneurysmal portions of the left ventricle (**c**–**f**).

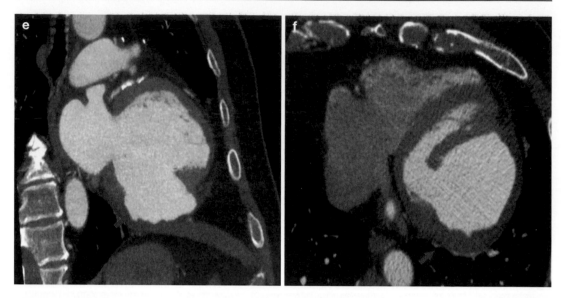

Fig. 5.8 (continued)

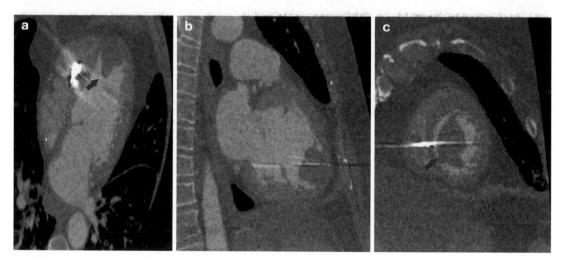

Fig. 5.9 (**a–c**) Multiplanar reformat images in the four-chamber, two-chamber, and short axis view demonstrate a large filling defect at the apex, consistent with a thrombus (*red arrow*)

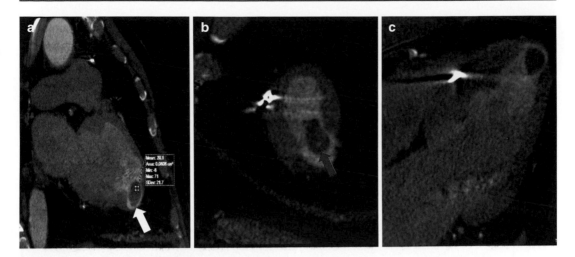

Fig. 5.10 (**a–c**) Multiplanar reformat images in the four-chamber, two-chamber, and short axis view demonstrate thinning of the myocardium due to an infarct (*white arrow*), also noted is a large filling defect at the apex within the aneurysmal apex, consistent with a thrombus (*red arrow*)

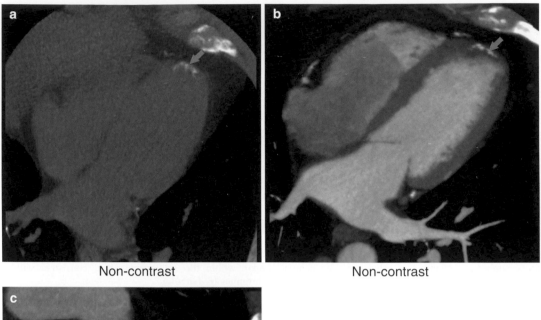

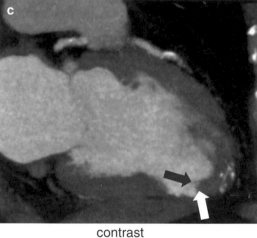

contrast

Fig. 5.11 (**a**) Axial noncontrast multiplanar reformat image demonstrates calcification at the apex of the left ventricle (*blue arrow*). Axial maximum intensity projection in the four-chamber (**b**) and two-chamber view (**c**) demonstrates left ventricular aneurysm (*white arrow*) with hypoattenuated region at the apex suggestive of thrombus, with curvilinear hyperdense area calcification (*blue arrow*) most consistent with a chronic thrombus (*red arrow*)

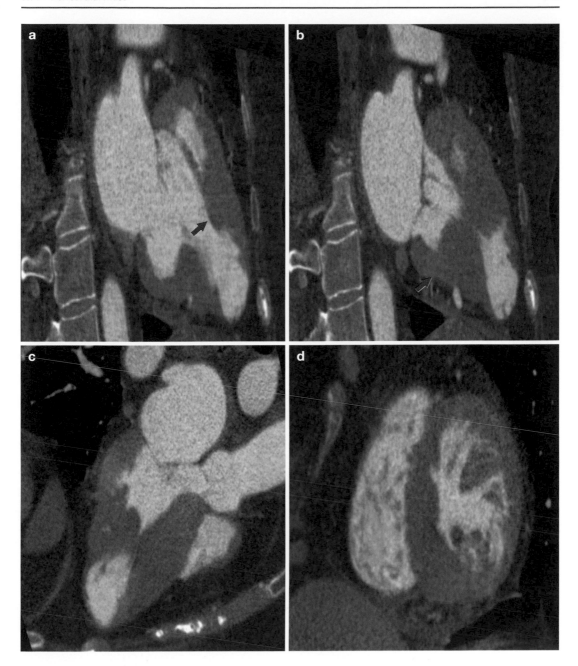

Fig. 5.12 Multiplanar reformatted images (**a**–**d**) demonstrate asymmetric hypertrophy of lateral left ventricular wall and the mid-segment of the interventricular septum (*red arrows*), with resultant left ventricular outflow tract obstruction. Note the sparing of the ventricular apex, which can be seen in HCM

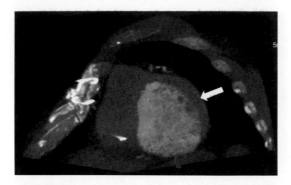

Fig 5.13 Maximum intensity projection in short axis demonstrates severe thinning of the inferior wall of the left ventricle (*red arrow*) secondary to prior myocardial infarction. The thin inferior left ventricle wall is in stark contrast with the normal myocardial thickness of the lateral wall of the left ventricle (*white arrow*).

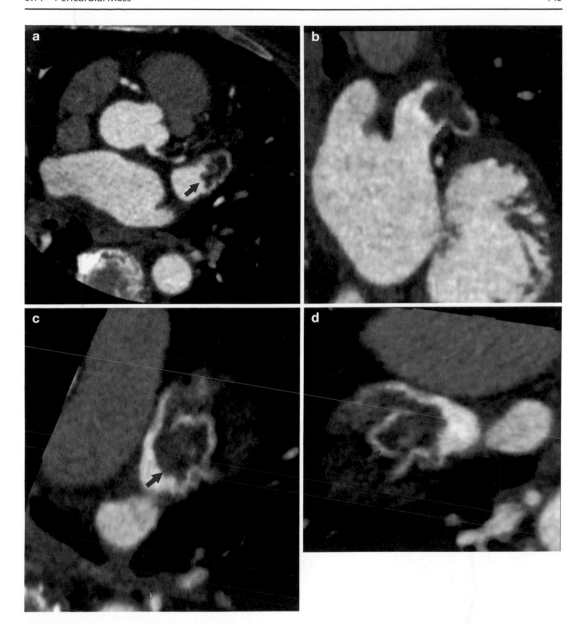

Fig. 5.14 Multiplanar reformat images in axial (**a**) and near two-chamber (**b**) views demonstrate a large filling defect (*red arrows*) in the left atrial appendage consistent with thrombus. Multiplanar reformatted images of the left atrium (**c**, **d**) demonstrate in detail the extent of the thrombus (*red arrows*). *Patients with atrial fibrillation have slow flow in the left atrial appendage ("smoke" on echo) leading to poor contrast filling which can mimic a thrombus. It is important to get delayed images to rule out thrombus*

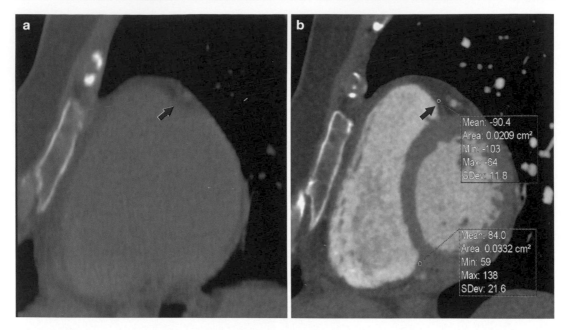

Fig. 5.15 Multiplanar reformat noncontrast (**a**) and contrast (**b**) images in short axis demonstrate patchy areas of hypoattenuation (*red arrow*) in the right ventricular wall, measuring fat density. The patient needs further workup with echo or cardiac MRI to evaluate for arrhythmogenic right ventricular cardiomyopathy (ARVC)

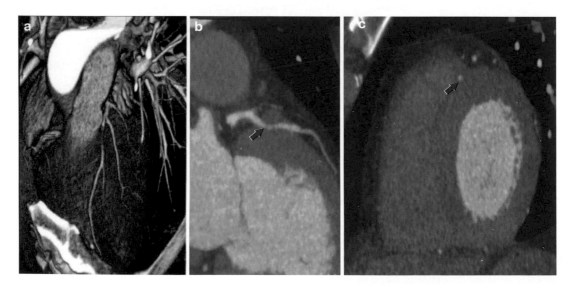

Fig. 5.16 (**a**) 3D volume rendered image in oblique sagittal view demonstrates myocardial bridge of mid LAD multiplanar. Maximum intensity projection in two-chamber (**b**) and short axis view (**c**) demonstrate a superficial bridging of the mid LAD (*red arrow*). It is important to evaluate the extent of bridging in a short axis view to accurately assess the depth of the bridge

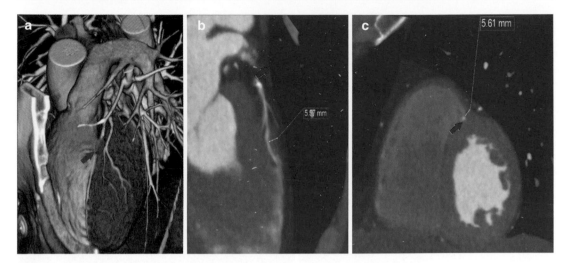

Fig. 5.17 (**a**) 3D volume rendered image in oblique sagittal view demonstrates myocardial bridge of mid LAD multiplanar. Maximum intensity projection in near two-chamber (**b**) and short axis (**c**) view demonstrates a deep bridging of the mid LAD (*red arrow*). Compare the depth of bridging with Fig. 5.16.

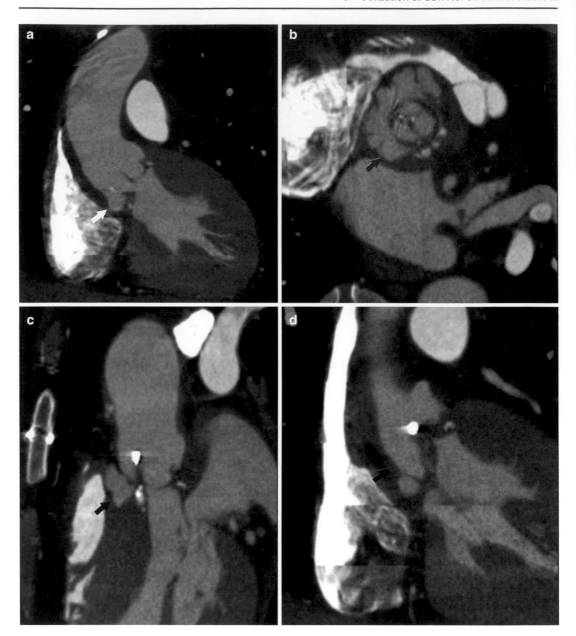

Fig. 5.18 Multiplanar CCTA (**a**) demonstrates abnormal soft tissue density (*white arrow*) along the aortic valve leaflet, representing vegetation, consistent with endocarditis. Multiplanar reformatted images (**b–d**) show abnormal fluid collection seen along the aortic root (*red arrow*) suspicious for aortic root abscess. There is an abnormal area filled with contrast adjacent to the aortic root (*blue arrows*), representing pseudoaneurysm

Aortic vegetation calcification

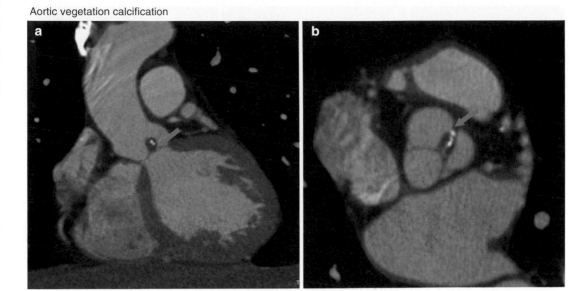

Fig. 5.19 Multiplanar reformat image in three-chamber (**a**) and cross-sectional view (**b**) of the aortic valve demonstrates a calcified soft tissue density (*blue arrows*) on the tip of the right and left coronary cusp, suggestive of vegetation

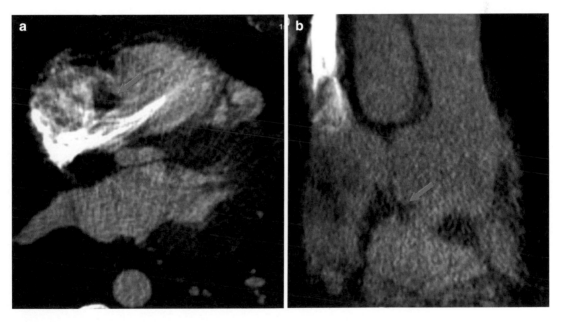

Fig. 5.20 Multiplanar reformat image in four-chamber (**a**) and right two-chamber (**b**) view demonstrates soft tissue density surrounding the tricuspid (*blue arrow*), suggestive of vegetation

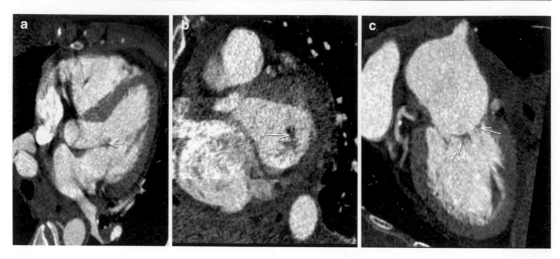

Fig. 5.21 Near four-chamber multiplanar reformatted image (**a**) demonstrates focal thickening measuring soft tissue attenuation (*white arrow*) of the mitral valve. Multiplanar CCTA (**b**, **c**) demonstrates soft tissue density surrounding the mitral valve leaflet (*white arrows*), suggestive of vegetation

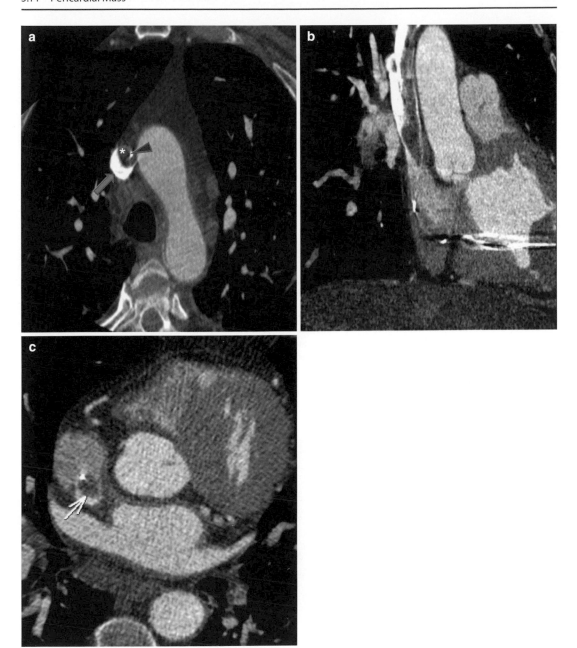

Fig. 5.22 (**a**) Axial multiplanar reformatted image at the level of aortic arch demonstrates a well-circumscribed hypoattenuated soft tissue density (*) in the superior vena cava (*blue arrow*) encircling the pacemaker lead (*arrowhead*), with high attenuating contrast extending circumferentially around it. Coronal multiplanar reformatted image (**b**) demonstrates well-circumscribed soft tissue density along the entire length of the pacemaker wire extending into right atrium, surrounded by contrast. Axial multiplanar reformatted image (**c**) at the level of aortic root demonstrates the soft tissue mass encircling pace maker lead (*white arrow*) in the right atrium. Given the patient's history of fever and positive blood cultures, this most likely represent infected thrombus/vegetation. In general, due to the relatively poor mixing that occurs in the superior vena cava from the laminar flow secondary to the entry of opacified blood from the right brachiocephalic vein (in this patient with right-sided IV contrast administration) and unopacified blood from the left brachiocephalic vein (and occasionally the azygous vein) a psuedothrombus appearance may occur. Delayed images will help increase diagnostic confidence

Left ventricle
hypoperfusion

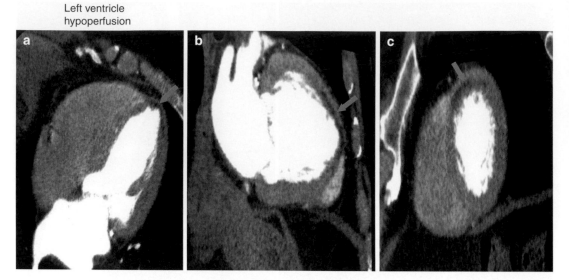

Fig. 5.23 Four-chamber multiplanar reformatted image (**a**) at rest demonstrate near-transmural hypoattenuation of the left ventricular apex (*blue arrow*) suggestive of at least resting hypoperfusion. Two-chamber multiplanar reformatted (**b**) and short axis (**c**) views demonstrate sub-endocardial low attenuation/hypoperfusion of the anterior wall of the left ventricle (*blue arrows*). Portions of the low hypoattenuation area of myocardium measure near fat-attenuation, which suggest an element of chronic infarct as well

Aortic annular calcification

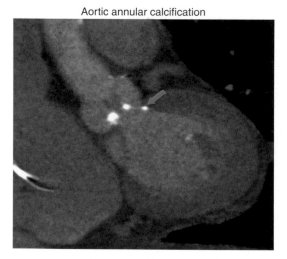

Fig. 5.24 Coronal three-chamber maximum intensity projection demonstrates focal aortic annular calcification. Also seen is calcification of the aortic valve leaflets

Aortic valve calcification

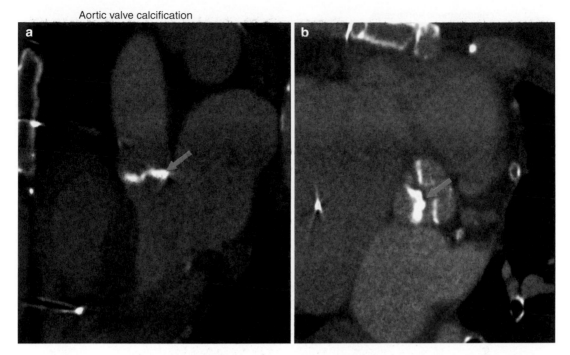

Fig. 5.25 Near three-chamber multiplanar reformatted image (**a**) demonstrates severe calcification of the aortic valve leaflets. En face multiplanar reformatted image (**b**) of the aortic valve demonstrates severe calcification, most severely affecting the noncoronary cusp

Aortic valve thickening with AL orifice

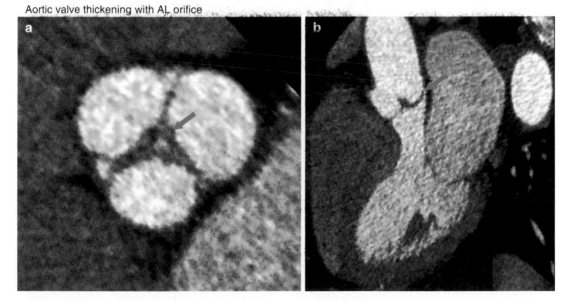

Fig. 5.26 En face multiplanar reformatted image (**a**) at the level of the aortic valve leaflets demonstrates noncalcified thickening of all three leaflets (*blue arrow*) with poor coaptation in diastole with resultant regurgitant ori-fice, which may be quantified. A three-chamber multiplanar reformatted image (**b**) demonstrates thickening (*blue arrow*)of the noncoronary cusp

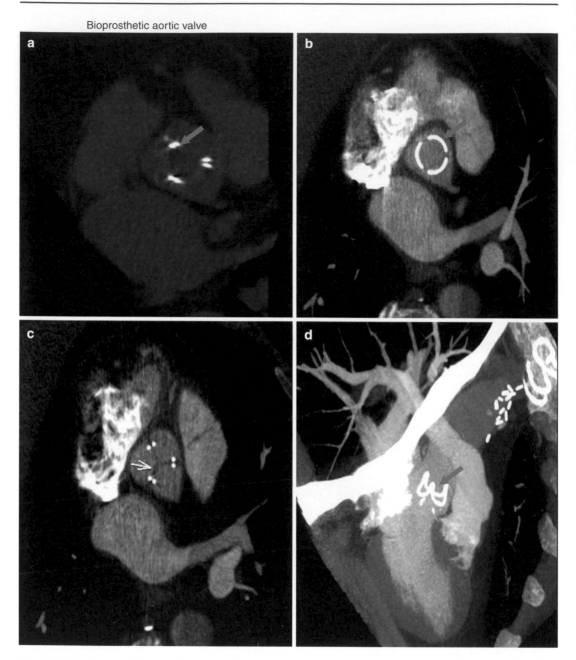

Fig. 5.27 En face multiplanar reformatted image of a bioprosthetic valve (**a**) in the aortic position demonstrates the struts of the three leaflets (*blue arrow*). En face images at the level of aortic root (**b**, **c**) demonstrates the three leaflets of a bioprosthetic valve (*blue arrows*) in the aortic position. The leaflets are thin, smooth, and completely coapt in diastole (*white arrow*). There is no evidence of regurgitant orifice or vegetation on this image. Three-chamber maximum intensity projection (**d**) demonstrates the three-dimensional nature of a bioprosthetic valve (*blue arrow*) in the mitral position

Mechanical aortic valve

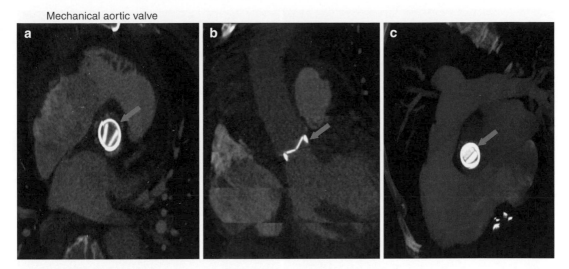

Fig. 5.28 En face image of the aortic annulus (**a–c**) demonstrates a mechanical valve, with its high attenuation frame and two semicircular high attenuating leaflets (*blue arrows*). The frame is in close apposition to the suture ring/aortic annulus complex – without evidence of dehiscence

Ebstein's anomaly repair

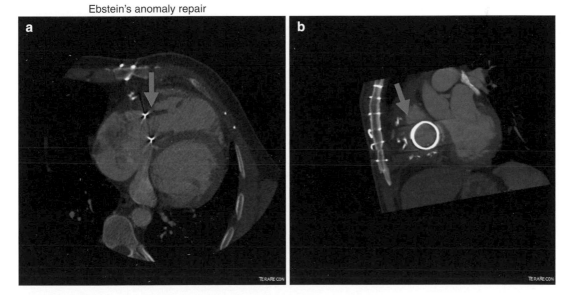

Fig. 5.29 Long axis two-chamber view (**a**) of the right ventricle demonstrates a bioprosthetic valve in the tricuspid position (*blue arrow*) in this patient status post Ebstein's anomaly repair. Left ventricular outflow tract view (**b**) demonstrates the right atrium and coronary sinus are dilated (*blue arrow*)

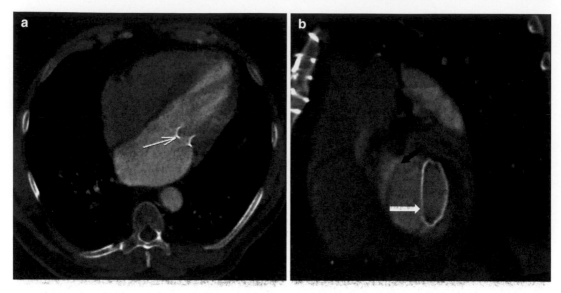

Fig. 5.30 Four-chamber (**a**) and short axis (**b**) multiplanar reformatted images demonstrate severe leftward displacement (*white arrow*) of the right aspect of a mitral annular ring into the lumen – diagnostic of annuloplasty ring dehiscence. Arrow in the short axis image (**b**) indicates the native mitral annulus

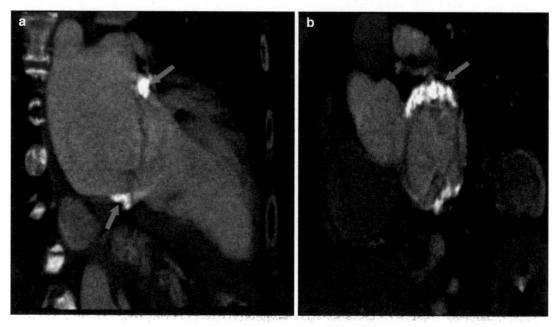

Fig. 5.31 Long axis two-chamber (**a**) and short axis (**b**) multiplanar reformatted images demonstrate bulky mitral annular calcification (*blue arrows*), most prominent anteriorly. The mitral valve leaflets are spared

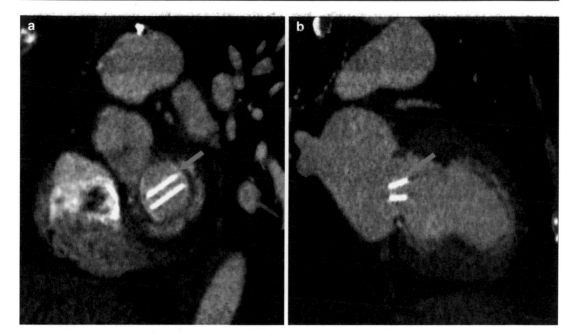

Fig. 5.32 Short axis (**a**) multiplanar reformation at the level of the mitral valve annulus in diastole demonstrates expected positioning of the mechanical mitral valve (*blue arrows*) without evidence of pannus or vegetation. Two-chamber long axis (**b**) multiplanar reformatted images demonstrate an intact suture ring/native mitral annulus complex (*blue arrows*) – without dehiscence or prominent pannus

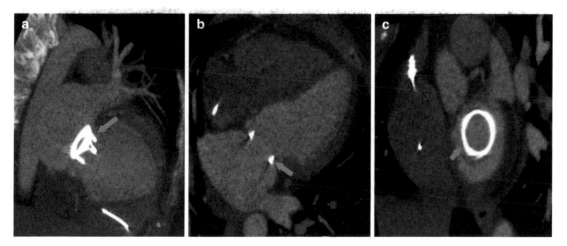

Fig. 5.33 (**a**) Long axis longitudinal two-chamber maximum intensity projection image demonstrates the three-dimensional nature of a bioprosthetic valve (*blue arrow*) in the mitral position. Four-chamber (**b**) multiplanar reformatted images demonstrate close apposition of the metallic stent/frame ring portion to the suture ring/native mitral annulus complex (*blue arrow*) – without gross dehiscence. Near short axis (**c**) multiplanar reformat demonstrates the circular metallic stent/frame in expected location (*blue arrow*)

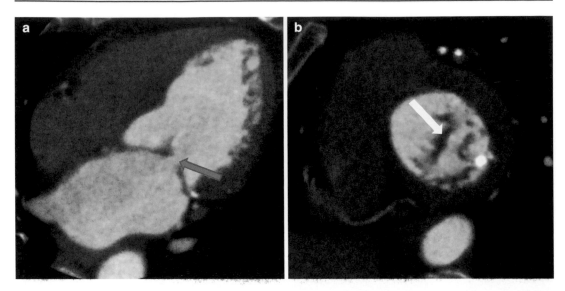

Fig. 5.36 (**a**, **b**) Multiplanar reformat image in four-chamber (**a**) and short axis (**b**) during diastole demonstrates thickened anterior and posterior mitral valve leaflets (*white arrow*) with a narrowed mitral valve orifice suspicious for an element of mitral stenosis, which should be confirmed with echocardiography (*blue arrow*)

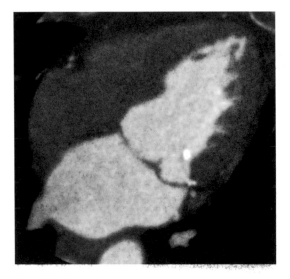

Fig. 5.37 Four-chamber multiplanar reformat image in systole demonstrates posterior/superior bowing of both the anterior and posterior leaflets mitral valve greater than 2 mm beyond the mitral annular plane, diagnostic of mitral valve prolapse

References

1. Aslam A, Khokar US, Chaudhry AA. Assessment of isotropic calcium using 0.5-mm reconstructions from 320-row CT data sets identifies more patients with non-zero Agatston score and more subclinical atherosclerosis than standard 3.0-mm coronary artery calcium scan and CT angiography. J Cardiovasc Comput Tomogr. 2014;8(1):58–66.

2. Poon M, Cortegiano M, et al. Associations between routine coronary computed tomographic angiography and reduced unnecessary hospital admissions, length of stay, recidivism rates, and invasive coronary angiography in the Emergency Department triage of chest pain. J Am Coll Cardiol. 2013;62(6):543–52.

3. Budoff MJ, Hokanson JE, Nasir K, et al. Progression of coronary artery calcium predicts all-cause mortality. JACC Cardiovasc Imaging. 2010;3:1229–36.

4. Nieman K, et al. Differentiation of recent and chronic myocardial infarction by cardiac computed tomography. Am J Cardiol. 2006;98(3):303–8.

5. Becker CR, Kleffel T, Crispin A, et al. Coronary artery calcium measurement: agreement of multirow detector and electron beam CT. Am J Roentgenol. 2001;176:1295–8.

6. Gerber BL, et al. Accuracy of contrast-enhanced magnetic resonance imaging in predicting improvement of regional myocardial function in patients after acute myocardial infarction. Circulation. 2002;106(9):1083–9.

7. Kim RJ, et al. Relationship of MRI delayed contrast enhancement to irreversible injury, infarct age, and contractile function. Circulation. 1999;100(19):1992–2002.

8. Hesse B, et al. Images in cardiovascular medicine. A left atrial appendage thrombus mimicking atrial myxoma. Circulation. 2006;113(11):e456–7.

9. Mohrs OK, et al. Percutaneous left atrial appendage transcatheter occlusion (PLAATO): planning and follow-up using contrast-enhanced MRI. AJR Am J Roentgenol. 2006;186(2):361–4.

10. Mohrs OK, et al. Thrombus detection in the left atrial appendage using contrast-enhanced MRI: a pilot study. AJR Am J Roentgenol. 2006;186(1):198–205.

11. Parekh A, et al. Images in cardiovascular medicine. The case of a disappearing left atrial appendage thrombus: direct visualization of left atrial thrombus migration, captured by echocardiography, in a patient with atrial fibrillation, resulting in a stroke. Circulation. 2006;114(13):e513–4.

12. Blackshear JL, et al. Stroke prevention in atrial fibrillation: warfarin faces its challengers. Curr Cardiol Rep. 2005;7(1):16–22.

13. Mutlu B, et al. Fibrillatory wave amplitude as a marker of left atrial and left atrial appendage function, and a predictor of thromboembolic risk in patients with rheumatic mitral stenosis. Int J Cardiol. 2003; 91(2–3):179–86.

14. Luk A, Ahn E, Soor GS, Butany J. Dilated cardiomyopathy: a review. J Clin Pathol. 2009;62:219.

15. Elliott P. Cardiomyopathy. Diagnosis and management of dilated cardiomyopathy. Heart. 2000;84:106.

16. Abbara S, et al. Pericardial and Myocardial disease. In: Miller SW, editor. Cardiac imaging the requisites. 2nd ed. Philadelphia: Mosby; 2005. p. 270–2.

17. Mestrioni L, et al. Dilated cardiomyopathies. In: Fuster V et al., editors. Hurst's the heart. 11th ed. New York: Mc Graw-Hill; 2004. p. 1889–907.

18. Felker CM, et al. Underlying causes and long-term survival in patients with initially unexplained cardiomyopathy. N Engl J Med. 2000;342:1077–84.

19. Cooke CE, et al. Idiopathic dilated cardiomyopathy. N Engl J Med. 1995;332:1384–6.

20. Dec GW, et al. Idiopathic dilated cardiomyopathy. N Engl J Med. 1994;331:1564–75.

21. Rochitte CE, et al. The emerging role of MRI in the diagnosis and management of cardiomyopathies. Curr Cardiol Rep. 2006;8(1):44–52.

22. Kantor B, et al. Good news on coronary computed tomographic angiography: answers that have questions. Eur Heart J. 2008;29(17):2070–2.

23. Choo KS, et al. Adenosine-stress low-dose single-scan CT myocardial perfusion imaging using a 128-slice dual-source CT: a comparison with fractional flow reserve. Acta Radiol. 2013;54:389–95.

24. Heatlie GL, et al. LV aneurysm: comprehensive assessment of morphology, structure and thrombus using cardiovascular MR. Clin Radiol. 2005;60(6): 687–92.

25. Konen E, et al. True versus false left ventricular aneurysm: differentiation with MR imaging–initial experience. Radiology. 2005;236(1):65–70.

26. Ha JW, et al. Left ventricular aneurysm after myocardial infarction. Clin Cardiol. 1998;21(12):917.

27. Buck T, et al. Tomographic three-dimensional echocardiographic determination of chamber size and systolic function in patients with left ventricular aneurysm: comparison to magnetic resonance imaging, cineventriculography, and two-dimensional echocardiography. Circulation. 1997;96(12):4286–97.

28. Nicolosi AC, et al. Quantitative analysis of regional systolic function with left ventricular aneurysm. Curr Surg. 1988;45(5):387–9.

29. Aguiar J, Barba M, et al. Left ventricular aneurysm and differential diagnosis with pseudoaneurysm. Rev Port Cardiol. 2012;31:459–62.

30. Korosoglou G, et al. Prompt resolution of an apical left ventricular thrombus in a patient with takotsubo cardiomyopathy. Int J Cardiol. 2007;116(3):e88–91.

31. Morlese JF, et al. Acute ventricular and aortic thrombosis post chemotherapy. Br J Radiol. 2007;80(952): e75–7.

32. Mueller J, et al. Cardiac CT angiography after coronary bypass surgery: prevalence of incidental findings. AJR Am J Roentgenol. 2007;189(2):414–9.

33. Rustemli A, et al. Evaluating cardiac sources of embolic stroke with MRI. Echocardiography. 2007; 24(3):301–8; discussion 308.

Procedural Complications

6

Muzammil H. Musani

This chapter is a compilation of some of the unique and interesting case presentations, which will emphasize on the utilization of cardiac computed tomographic angiography when dealing with procedural complications.

Case 1

A 55-year-old asymptomatic patient was referred to our emergency department after a routine left subclavian venous port preremoval chest radiograph demonstrated a fractured fragment of the indwelling catheter in the left apical region. A nongated chest CT without contrast failed to precisely reveal location of the embolized fractured distal fragment in the right heart. A transthoracic echocardiogram failed to demonstrate the catheter fragment. An initial attempt to percutaneously remove the embolized fractured fragment using a snare catheter was unsuccessful. A prospectively triggered EKG-gated cardiac CTA was performed, which revealed the fractured catheter fragment lodged in the coronary sinus. The body of the catheter traversed across the tricuspid valve with the tip of the other end abutting the RV free wall. With the precise location of the entrapped catheter identified, the fragment was easily removed by looping a pigtail catheter around the mid portion of the catheter. The superb spatial and temporal resolution of EKG-gated cardiac CTA greatly facilitates preprocedural planning.

M.H. Musani et al., *Clinical Pearls in Diagnostic Cardiac Computed Tomographic Angiography*,
DOI 10.1007/978-3-319-08168-7_6, © Springer International Publishing Switzerland 2015

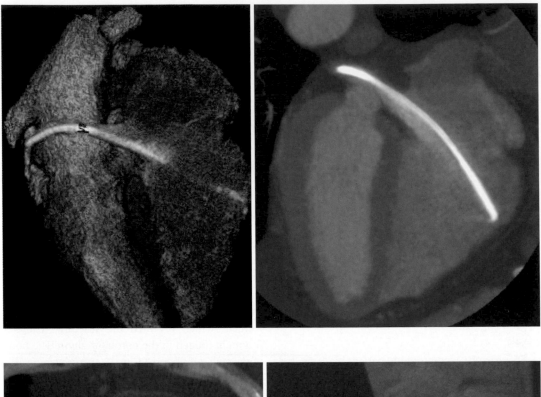

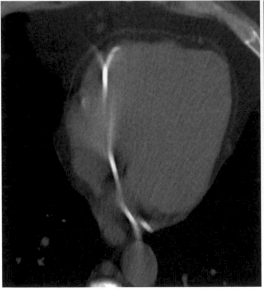

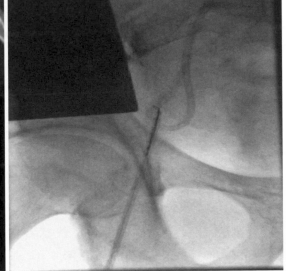

Case 2

A 32-year-old man with a history of remote right femur fracture presented to the emergency department complaining of dyspnea and sharp chest pain. Initial vital signs demonstrated tachycardia with 104 bpm. CT pulmonary angiogram and transthoracic echocardiogram demonstrated findings suggestive of hemopericardium with tamponade physiology, which was confirmed and treated with pericardiocentesis. Subsequent EKG-gated cardiac CT revealed three identical 2.3 cm linear metallic objects in the following locations: (1) perforating and lodged in the right ventricle free wall (*Black arrow*), (2) right ventricular cavity (*Blue Arrow*), and (3) right lower lobe (*White arrow*). Further patient questioning revealed a history of irretrievable inferior vena cava filter placement at the time of his femur fracture 10 years ago. An abdominal CT revealed an IVC filter missing three of its "arms (*Blue, white and black arrows*)." The patient was subsequently managed without surgical intervention and is being closely monitored.

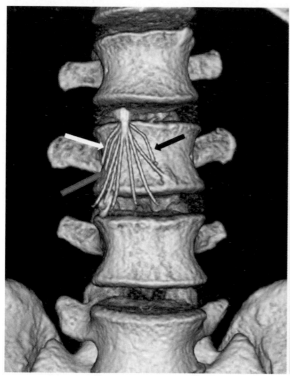
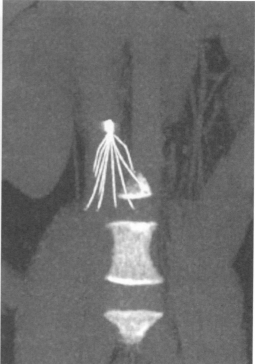
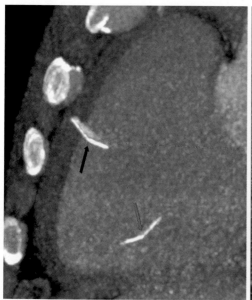
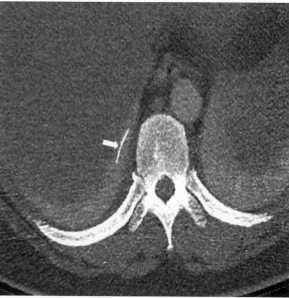

Case 3

A 58-year-old male with no past medical history and a remote history of mitral ring annuloplasty presents to the emergency department with complains of chest pain on exertion. Cardiac CTA revealed total occlusion of left circumflex in close proximity to the mitral annular ring (*white arrow*). Collateralization with robust contrast filling of the circumflex branches suggests chronicity (*arrow heads*). Remaining coronary arteries were normal.

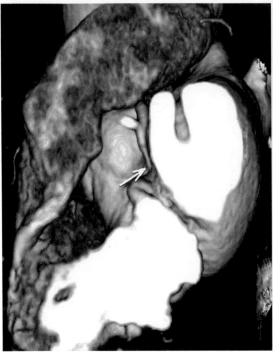 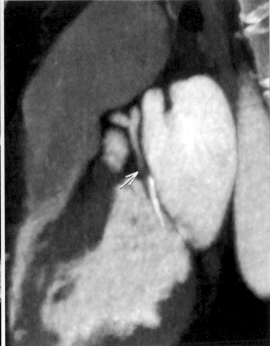

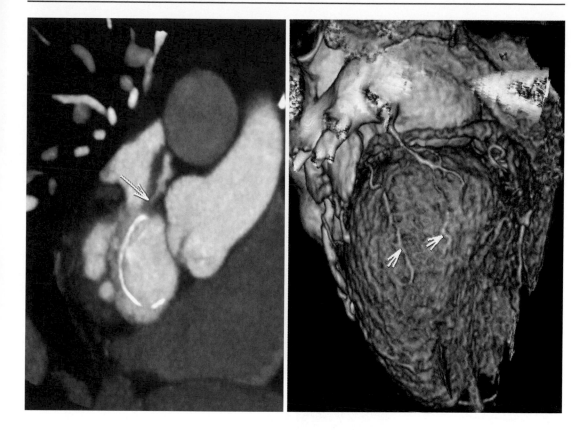

Case 4

A 62-year-old female with a remote history of metallic mitral valve replacement underwent placement of biventricular pacemaker. During the procedure the multiple attempts to place the wire in the coronary sinus (*blue arrow*) failed. The patient had a cardiac CTA which revealed occluded coronary sinus (*white arrow*) in the close proximity of the mitral valve annular ring suggestive of iatrogenic suturing of the coronary sinus.

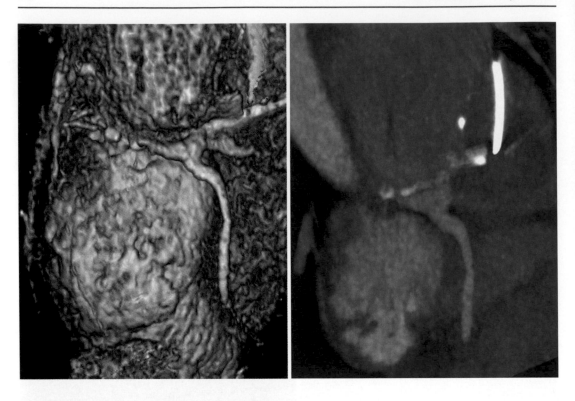

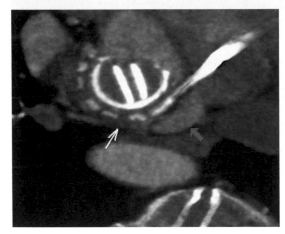

Case 5

A 68-year-old female with a history of distal obstructive LAD underwent minimally invasive robotic assist coronary artery bypass graft, LIMA to mid LAD. The patient was complaining of postoperative chest pressure. Troponins were trending up and echo reveal left ventricular anterior wall-motion abnormality. Cardiac CTA revealed a patent LIMA graft to mid LAD; however, there was no flow in the distal LAD. These findings are suggestive of grafting of the LIMA proximal to the obstructive lesion in the mid LAD.

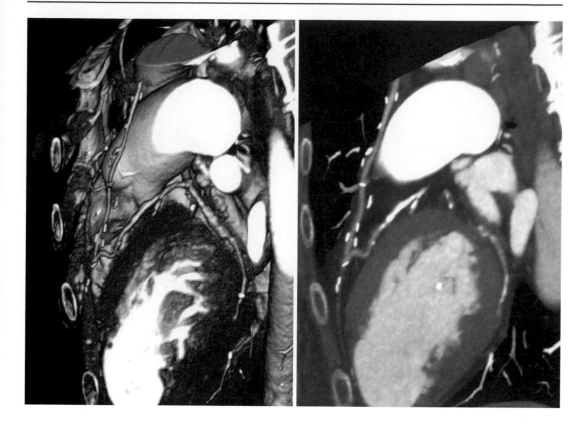

Case 6

A 48-year-old male who presented to the emergency department with chest pain was found to have NSTEMI. The patient underwent an urgent cardiac catheterization which was complicated by left main dissection. Cardiac CTA later revealed pseudoaneurysm of the left main coronary artery with thrombus (*Red Arrow*).

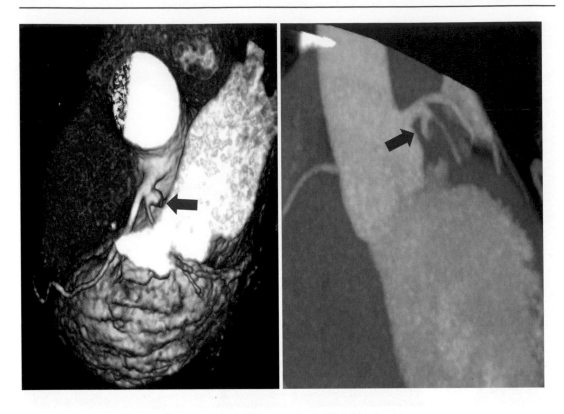

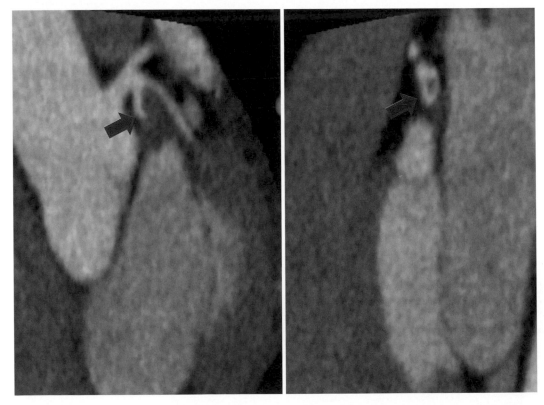

Case 7

A 69-year-old male with a recent history of left atrial ablation for atrial fibrillation develops shortness of breath on exertion for 1 month.

Cardiac CTA revealed greater than 70 % decrease in cross-sectional diameter of the right upper lobe pulmonary vein (RUPV) *White Arrow*.

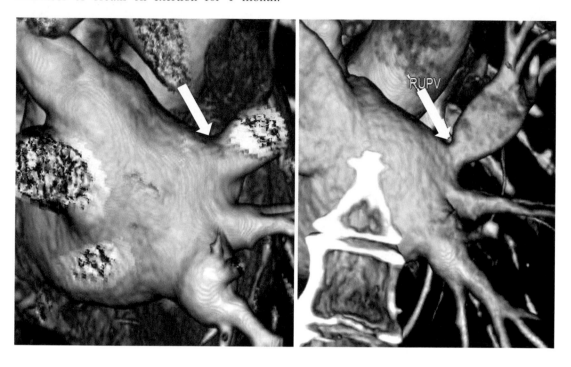

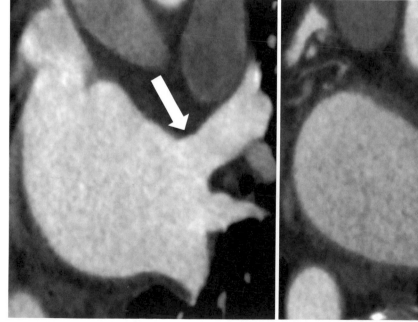

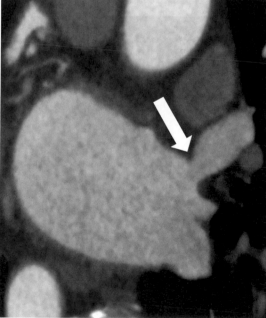

Pre-ablation   Post-ablation

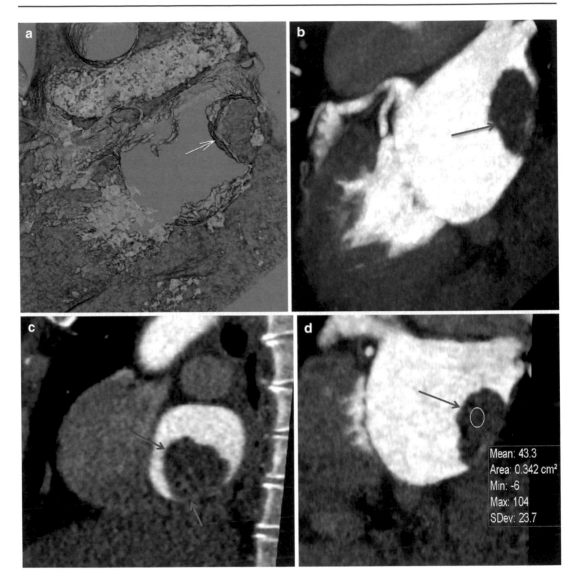

Fig. 7.1 (**a**) A two-chamber hollow volume rendered image demonstrates a large mass adhered to the left atrial wall (*white arrow*). (**b**) Maximum intensity projection near two-chamber image demonstrates a well-circumscribed, lobulated, pedunculated mass within the left atrium which extends from the inferior atrial wall in a sessile configuration (*red arrow*). (**c**) An oblique-sagittal MPR view demonstrate the mild heterogeneous enhancement at the base (*blue arrow*). (**d**) Coronal reconstructed image demonstrates the mass *to have a soft tissue attenuation of 43.3 HU*. These findings are diagnostic of left atrial myxoma

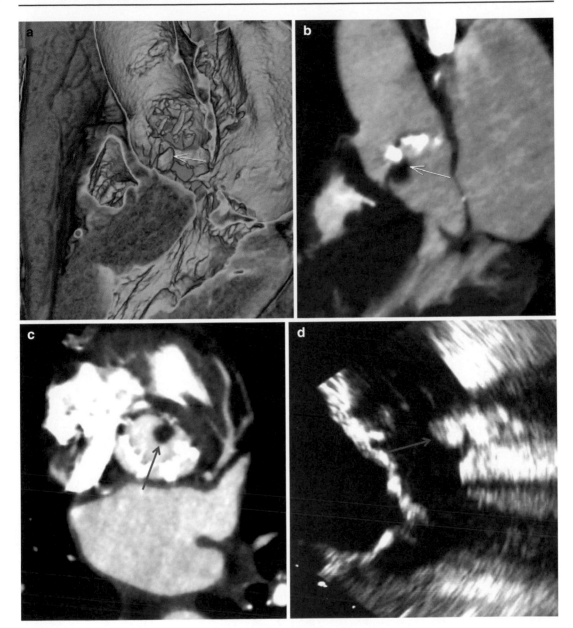

Fig. 7.2 (**a, b**) Hollow volume rendered image and maximum intensity projection image in a near three chamber view demonstrates a pedunculated mass on the ventricular aspect of the aortic valve leaflet (*white arrows*). (**c**) Multiplanar reformatted cross sectional image of the aortic valve demonstrates the mass which is consistent with a fibroelastoma. There is a pedunculated round mass juxtra-positioned to the coronary cusp (*red arrow*). (**d**) Echocardiogram which demonstrates a round, pendunculated, relatively hyper-echoic mass juxtapositioned to an aortic valve leaflet (*red arrow*). *Note that the soft tissue attenuation of this mass excludes a lipoma.*

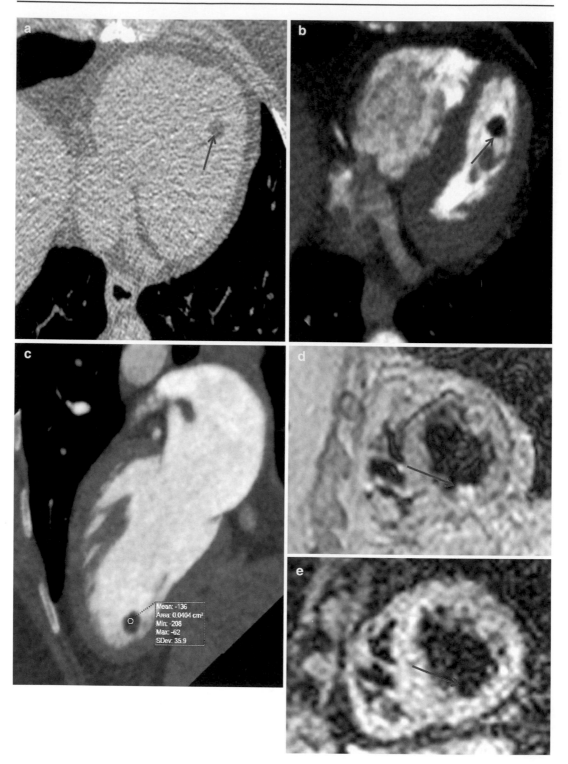

Fig. 7.3 (**a**) Axial non contrast image of the heart demonstrating a relatively hypoattenuating mass within the left ventricle (*red arrow*). (**b**) On the contrast portion of the study, the mass appears to be juxtapositioned to the papillary muscles, and is relatively hypoattenuating when compared to the adjacent myocardium (*red arrow*); (**c**) *sagittal reconstruction of the same patient with an ROI (region of interest) over the mass demonstrates a fatty attenuation of -136 HU (red arrow).* (**d**) T1 weighted image in short axis demonstrates a focal hyper-intense lesion with in the papillary muscles (*red arrow*). (**e**) T1 weighted fat saturated image in short axis at the same level; notice the signal drop out of the lesion (*red arrow*). These findings are diagnostic for intra papillary lipoma.

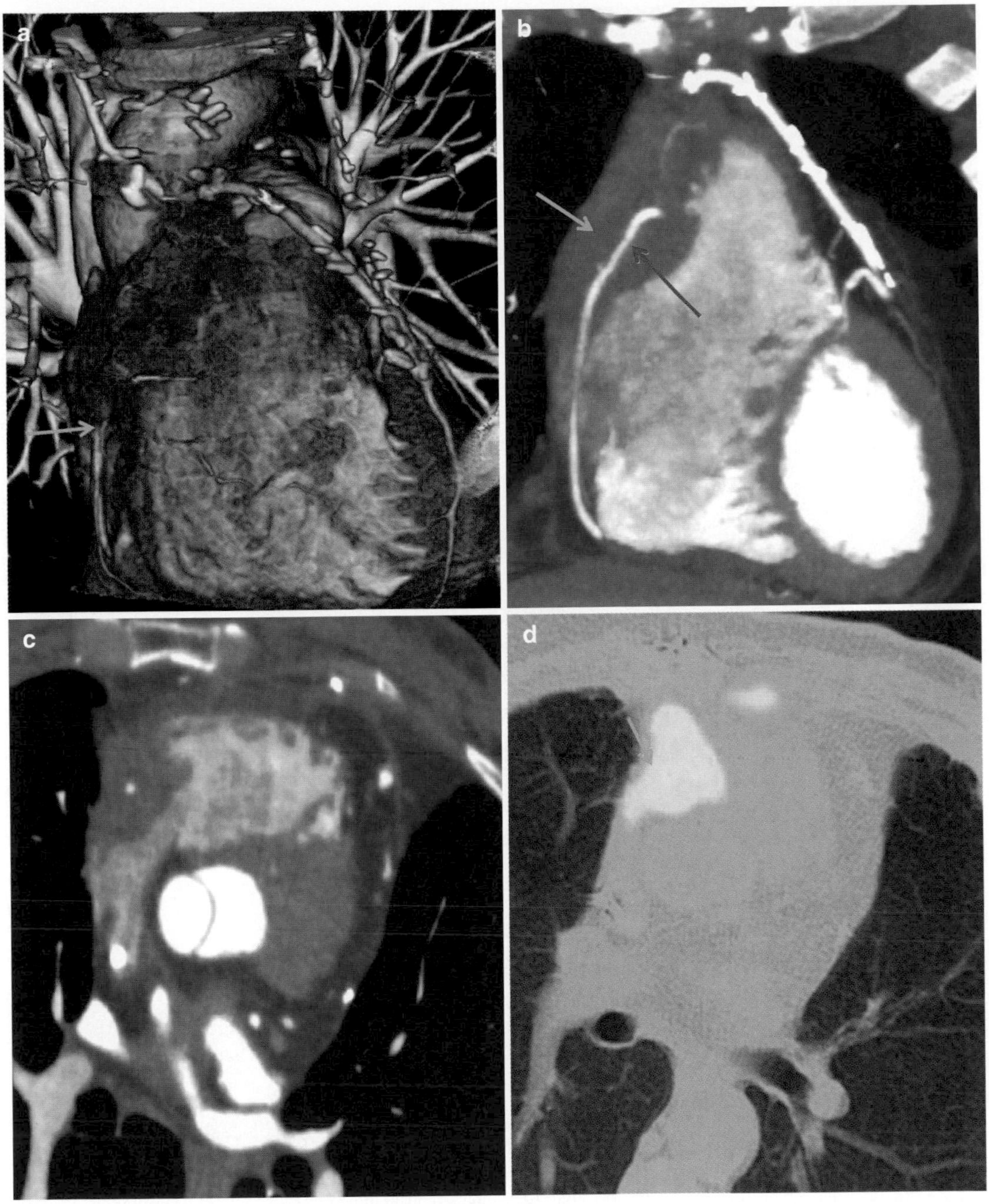

Fig. 7.4 (**a**) Volume rendered image in coronal plane demonstrates a mass within the outer wall of the right atrium (*green arrows*). (**b**) A coronal contrast-enhanced MIP (maximal intensity projection) of the same patient which demonstrates the mass (*red arrow*) in the outer wall of the right atrium; notice that it circumferentially encases the RCA (*green arrow*). (**c**) Maximum intensity projection axial image of the same patient demonstrate the mass (*red arrow*) as it encases the RCA (*green arrow*). (**d**) *PET-CT which demonstrates hypermetabolic activity correlating to the site of the mass on the other images.* This patient has a history of metastatic breast carcinoma; therefore, this likely represents a metastasis

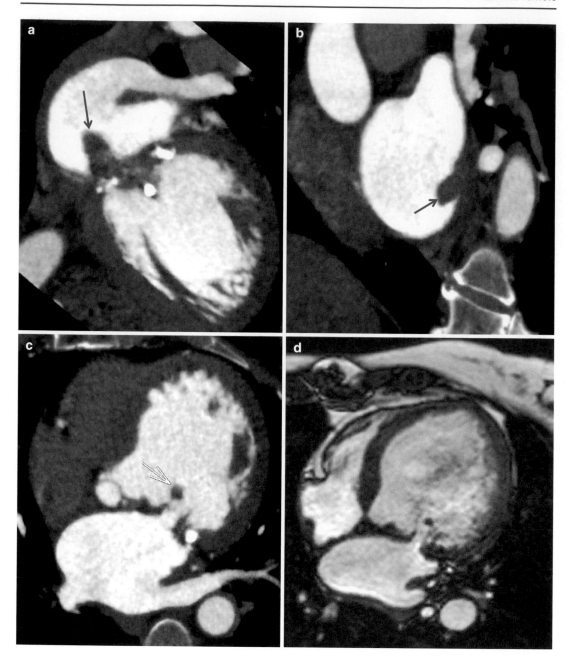

Fig. 7.5 (**a**) Coronal reconstructed image of a contrast-enhanced CT of the chest which demonstrates a frond like mass projecting off the mitral valve into the left atrium (*red arrow*). *This mass has a soft tissue density and is originating from the mitral valve annulus, at the site of a bioprosthetic valve. This represents a pannus.* (**b**) Oblique coronal view of the patient which demonstrates the pannus extending into the left atrial lumen (*red arrow*). (**c**) Axial contrast image of the same patient which demonstrates pedunculated vegetation extending into the left ventricle during diastole (*white arrow*). (**d**) An axial bright blood steady state free precession (SSFP) sequence of the heart which demonstrates that same small vegetation shown on (**c**) projecting into the left ventricular lumen during diastole (*red arrow*)

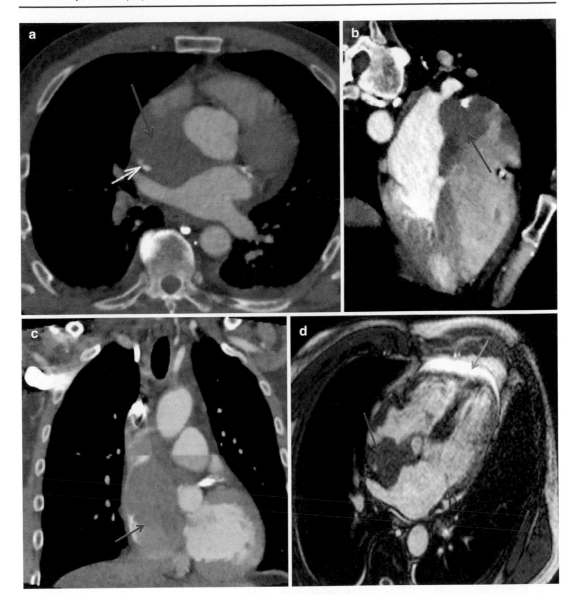

Fig. 7.6 (**a**) A contrast-enhanced axial CT image of a patient with cardiac lymphoma. Notice the infiltrative mass involving both the right atrial myocardium and lumen (*red arrow*). Note how the mass involves the right AV groove and encases a portion of the RCA (*white arrow*). (**b**) A slightly oblique axial image demonstrating the long axis of the heart, also demonstrating the lymphomatous mass in the right atrium (*red arrow*) with encasement of the RCA (*green arrow*). (**c**) A coronal reformatted image of the same patient demonstrating the lymphomatous mass involving both the right atrial myocardium and lumen (*red arrow*). (**d**) A fluid sensitive axial sequence of the heart demonstrating an irregular lymphomatous mass involving the interatrial septum (*red arrow*). Notice the associated pericardial effusion demonstrated by a crescent of hyperintense signal surrounding the apex of the heart (*green arrow*)

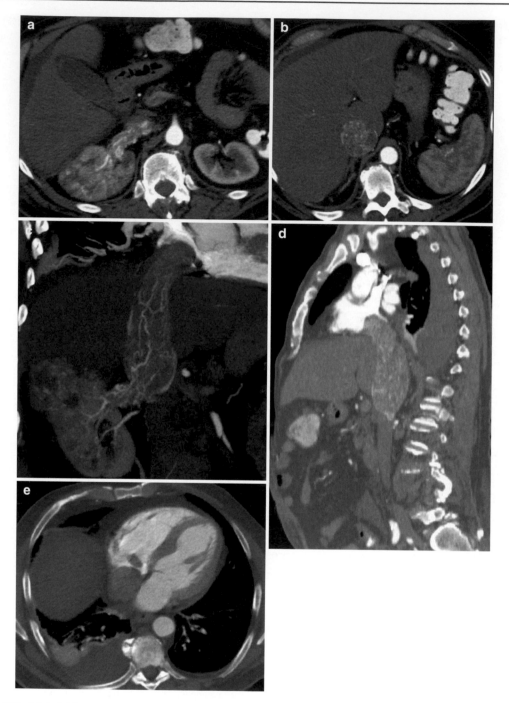

Fig. 7.7 (a) Axial image in venous phase demonstrates a very bizarre, heterogeneous pattern of enhancement involving the entire right kidney with extension into the right renal vein (*red arrow*). (b) axial image in the venous phase at the level of intra hepatic inferior vena cava demonstrates a heterogeneously enhancing mass completely occupying the inferior vena cava (*red arrow*). (c) Oblique coronal image in venous phase demonstrates diffuse infiltration and heterogeneous enhancement of the right kidney (*blue arrow*) with extension into the right renal vein (*green arrow*). This also extends cephalad through the IVC to involve the right atrium (*red arrows*). (d–e) Sagittal and axial images demonstrates the heterogeneously enhancing, circumscribed mass within the IVC extending cephalad to involve the right atrium (*red arrows*). These findings are consistent with renal cell carcinoma with tumor thrombus extending into the IVC and right atrium.

References

1. Lam KY, Dickens P, Chan AC. Tumors of the heart. A 20-year experience with a review of 12,485 consecutive autopsies. Arch Pathol Lab Med. 1993;117:1027.
2. McAllister Jr, H.A. Tumors of the cardiovascular system. In: Atlas of tumor pathology, second. Washington, DC: Armed Forces Institute of Pathology; 1978. Vol Fascicle 15.
3. Salcedo EE, Cohen GI, White RD, Davison MB. Cardiac tumors: diagnosis and management. Curr Probl Cardiol. 1992;17:73.
4. Silvestri F, Bussani R, Pavletic N, Mannone T. Metastases of the heart and pericardium. G Ital Cardiol. 1997;27:1252.
5. Cortan Ramzi S, Kumar V, Collins T, Robbins SL. The heart. In : Pathologic basis of disease. 6th ed. Philadelphia: Saunders; 1999. P. 543–99. Print.
6. Vander Salm TJ. Unusual primary tumors of the heart. Semin Thorac Cardiovasc Surg. 2000;12:89.
7. Elbardissi AW, Dearani JA, Daly RC, et al. Embolic potential of cardiac tumors and outcome after resection: a case–control study. Stroke. 2009;40:156.
8. Lee VH, Connolly HM, Brown Jr RD. Central nervous system manifestations of cardiac myxoma. Arch Neurol. 2007;64:1115.
9. Kuon E, Kreplin M, Weiss W, Dahm JB. The challenge presented by right atrial myxoma. Herz. 2004; 29:702.
10. ElBardissi AW, Dearani JA, Daly RC, et al. Analysis of benign ventricular tumors: long-term outcome after resection. J Thorac Cardiovasc Surg. 2008;135:1061.
11. Keeling IM, Oberwalder P, Anelli-Monti M, et al. Cardiac myxomas: 24 years of experience in 49 patients. Eur J Cardiothorac Surg. 2002;22:971.
12. Jelic J, Milicić D, Alfirević I, et al. Cardiac myxoma: diagnostic approach, surgical treatment and follow-up. A twenty years experience. J Cardiovasc Surg (Torino). 1996;37:113.
13. Pinede L, Duhaut P, Loire R. Clinical presentation of left atrial cardiac myxoma. A series of 112 consecutive cases. Medicine (Baltimore). 2001;80:159.
14. Alrashdi I, Bano G, Maher ER, Hodgson SV. Carney triad versus Carney Stratakis syndrome: two cases which illustrate the difficulty in distinguishing between these conditions in individual patients. Fam Cancer. 2010;9:443.
15. O'Donnell DH, et al. Cardiac tumors: optimal cardiac MR sequences and spectrum of imaging appearances. AJR Am J Roentgenol. 2009;193(2):377–87.
16. Grebnec ML, et al. Cardiac myxoma: imaging features in 83 patients. Radiographics. 2002;22(3):673–89.
17. Araoz PA, et al. CT and MR imaging of benign primary cardiac neoplasms with echocardiographic correlation. Radiographics. 2000;20(5):1303–19.
18. Gowda RM, Khan IA, Nair CK, et al. Cardiac papillary fibroelastoma: a comprehensive analysis of 725 cases. Am Heart J. 2003;146:404.
19. Sun JP, Asher CR, Yang XS, et al. Clinical and echocardiographic characteristics of papillary fibroelastomas: a retrospective and prospective study in 162 patients. Circulation. 2001;103:2687.
20. Grebenc ML, et al. Primary cardiac and pericardial neoplasms: radiologic-pathologic correlation. Radiographics. 2000;20(4):1073–103.
21. Edwards FH, et al. Primary cardiac valve tumors. Ann Thorac Surg. 1991;52(5):1127–31.
22. Matsushita T, et al. Aortric valve lipoma. Ann Thorac Surg. 2007;83(6):2220–2.
23. Gaerte SC, et al. Fat-containing lesions of the chest. Radiographics. 2002;22 Spec No: s61–78.
24. Vander Salm TJ, et al. Unusual primary tumors of the heart. Semin Thorac Cardiovac Surg. 2000;12(2):89–100.
25. Colucci WS, et al. Primary tumors of the heart. In: Braunwald E, editor. Heart disease: a textbook of cardiovascular medicine. 6th ed. Philadelphia: W.B. Saunders Company; 2001.
26. Benvenuti LA, Mansur AJ, Lopes DO, Campos RV. Primary lipomatous tumors of the cardiac valves. South Med J. 1996;89:1018.
27. Hananouchi GI, Goff 2nd WB. Cardiac lipoma: six-year follow-up with MRI characteristics, and a review of the literature. Magn Reson Imaging. 1990;8:825.
28. Caralps JM, Martí V, Ferrés P, et al. Mitral valve repair after excision of a fibrolipoma. Ann Thorac Surg. 1998;66:1808.
29. Burke AP, Cowan D, Virmani R. Primary sarcomas of the heart. Cancer. 1992;69:387.
30. Donsbeck AV, Ranchere D, Coindre JM, et al. Primary cardiac sarcomas: an immunohistochemical and grading study with long-term follow-up of 24 cases. Histopathology. 1999;34:295.
31. Simpson L, Kumar SK, Okuno SH, et al. Malignant primary cardiac tumors: review of a single institution experience. Cancer. 2008;112:2440.
32. Orlandi A, Ferlosio A, Roselli M, et al. Cardiac sarcomas: an update. J Thorac Oncol. 2010;5:1483.
33. Jeudy J, et al. From the radiologic-pathology archives: cardiac lymphoma: radiologic-pathologic correlation. Radiographics. 2012;32:1369–80.

Vascular Angiography

8

James Shin and Muzammil H. Musani

Arterial phase contrast studies, in particular when combined with multi-detector row CT capabilities, provide a highly useful diagnostic imaging tool for the evaluation of a multitude of vascular pathologies. In this chapter, we review in brief the epidemiology of several important angiographic diagnoses, and the clinical relevance of the pathophysiology underlying these clinical entities.

8.1 Aortic Aneurysm

The prevalence and incidence of thoracic aneurysms are difficult to ascertain accurately. As degenerative and atherosclerotic changes underlie most thoracic aortic aneurysms, the natural history is slowly progressive in the majority of cases. Genetic or inflammatory etiologies more commonly affect the thoracic rather than abdominal aorta. In two population studies [1, 2], annual incidence of thoracic aortic aneurysm was estimated to be 5.6 and 10.4 cases per 100,000 patient-years, likely an underestimation of true incidence as many such aneurysms are asymptomatic. Symptomatic thoracic aortic aneurysms are typically very large (5–6 cm or greater) and at increased risk for rupture.

Abdominal aortic aneurysms occur more commonly than the thoracic counterpart. Large-scale population screening studies demonstrate a prevalence of 4–8 % among elderly males, with increased risk of abdominal aortic aneurysm with advanced age, male gender, smoking, among other factors [3]. The majority of cases involve the infrarenal aorta, with approximately 5 % of cases involving the pararenal or suprarenal aorta. One retrospective analysis [4] of outpatients with abdominal aortic aneurysms found concomitant thoracic aortic aneurysm in approximately 25 % of subjects, with evidence of increased prevalence of comorbid thoracic aortic aneurysm in women; individually, thoracic and abdominal aneurysms have a male preponderance. Risk of rupture increases with aneurysm size and rate of growth, with larger aneurysm expanding at an increased rate [3–5].

8.2 Aortic Dissection

The primary event in acute aortic dissection is an intimal tear, leading to the characteristic intimal flap apparent on contrast-enhanced imaging studies. Propagation of the flap leads to extension of the dissection plane and creation of a false lumen, which can occlude branch vessels (e.g., coronary arteries) if the origin is compromised. The incidence of acute aortic dissection has been estimated to range from 2.6 to 3.5 cases per 100,000 person-years, with hypertension identified as one of the primary risk factors [6, 7]. Acute type A dissection (ascending aorta) is twice as common as type B (descending), and surgical management of this more frequently fatal subtype is preferred, whereas medical management is the mainstay of type B dissection not at risk of impending rupture [8].

M.H. Musani et al., *Clinical Pearls in Diagnostic Cardiac Computed Tomographic Angiography*, DOI 10.1007/978-3-319-08168-7_8, © Springer International Publishing Switzerland 2015

8.3   Coarctation

Coarctation of the aorta is defined as hemodynamically significant narrowing of the descending aorta, typically at the level of the ductus arteriosus insertion just distal to the origin of the left subclavian artery, distinguishing this entity from pseudo-coarctation, which is kinking or buckling of the descending aorta without hemodynamic compromise. Coarctation is estimated to be prevalent in approximately 4 per 10,000 live births, accounting for 4–6 % of all congenital heart defects [9, 10].

8.4   Patent Ductus Arteriosus

Half of term infants undergo ductal closure within the first 24 h after birth, virtually all within 72 h [11]. Delay in closure is inversely proportional to gestational age, and as a result of improvements in neonatal intensive care, the incidence of patent ductus arteriosus has increased [10]. Among term infants, incidence has been estimated between 0.03 and 0.08 % when defined as patency beyond six weeks. Sibling and family studies have demonstrated a genetic predisposition, although no specific genetic marker has been identified [9–12]. The myriad and dynamic effects of this congenital shunt have been well described, and are beyond the scope of this chapter.

8.5   Pulmonary Embolus

This common and often fatal clinical entity is the cause for significant morbidity and mortality (approximately 30 % when untreated) for a large number of patients. Previously, large-scale analyses have estimated the incidence of pulmonary embolus to be 1.5 % from all-cause mortality data, likely a significant underestimation as a large portion of subclinical pulmonary embolus remain undiagnosed [13, 14]. The advent and widespread use of CT angiography has allowed for improved diagnostic sensitivity, and newer data estimate incidence from 62 to 112 cases per 100,000 [14, 15].

8.6   Subclavian Steal

Reversal of flow within a vertebral artery ipsilateral to a hemodynamically significant proximal subclavian artery stenosis is most often an asymptomatic physiologic response to arterial disease. When symptomatic from vertebrobasilar insufficiency or, less commonly, limb ischemia; subclavian steal syndrome is manifest [16]. In a prospective cohort study of patients with asymptomatic neck bruits, 9 % were found with severe subclavian stenosis, and of these patients 64 % were found with subclavian steal syndrome – all with symptoms of vertebrobasilar insufficiency [17]. In a more recent large-scale prospective study [18], 6.5 % of patients undergoing carotid duplex scans were found with significant right/left arm pressure differential, with complete (persistent) steal occurring in 61 % of those patients. Only a small percentage of those with steal were symptomatic, again overwhelmingly from vertebrobasilar insufficiency. 7 of 38 symptomatic patients underwent intervention.

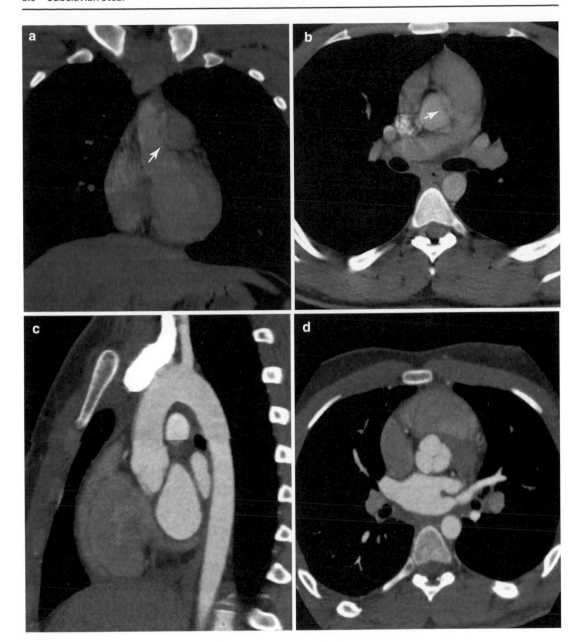

Fig. 8.1 Nongated aortogram in coronal (**a**) and axial (**b**) planes, demonstrating an apparent intimal flap (*white arrows*) at the aortic root, similar in appearance to aortic dissection. *This artifact is due to cardiac and aortic motion, and absence of a true dissection can be confirmed with an appropriately timed, gated study.* Gated aortogram in sagittal (**c**) and axial (**d**) planes in the same patient, obtained to rule out aortic dissection artifactually suggested from the prior figure. Although multi-detector technique allows for exceptionally fast volumetric acquisition, this advantage is not fully realized without gated coordination, capturing images free of motion during the cardiac cycle. *Furthermore, multiplanar evaluation is critical to distinguish valve leaflet from luminal flap, which can have similar appearance especially on the axial plane*

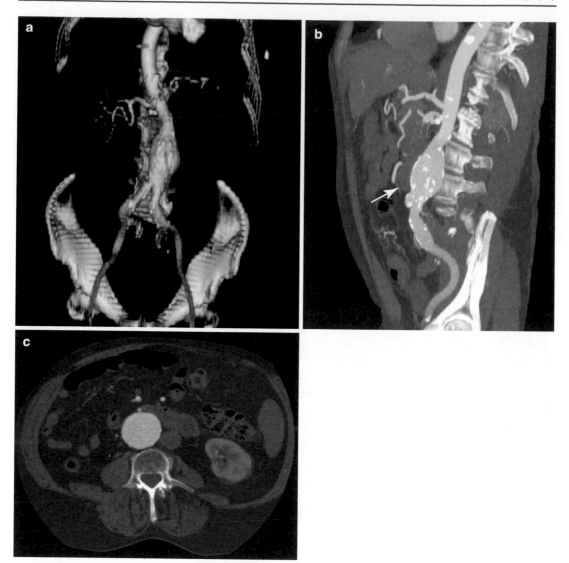

Fig. 8.2 3D volume rendered (**a**), sagittal maximum intensity projection (**b**), and axial (**c**) reconstructions demonstrating aneurysmal dilatation of the infrarenal aorta. Aortic diameter is normally up to 1.5 cm, with increasing risk of rupture with increasing size and/or rate of growth. Additionally noted is a small luminal out-pouching along the anteroinferior aspect, compatible with an ulcerated plaque (*white arrow*). *The presence of calcified plaque along the wall of the ulcer assists in identifying this coincident entity*

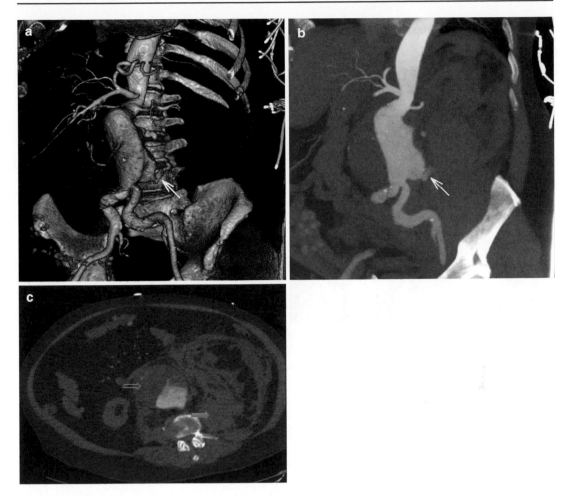

Fig. 8.3 3D volume rendered (**a**), sagittal maximum intensity projection (**b**), and axial (**c**) reconstructions demonstrating contrast extravasation along the posterior wall of an aneurysmal infrarenal aorta (*white arrow*), resulting in a large retroperitoneal hematoma (*blue arrow*). Note the smooth anterior luminal wall is delineated by a large thrombus (*black arrow*)

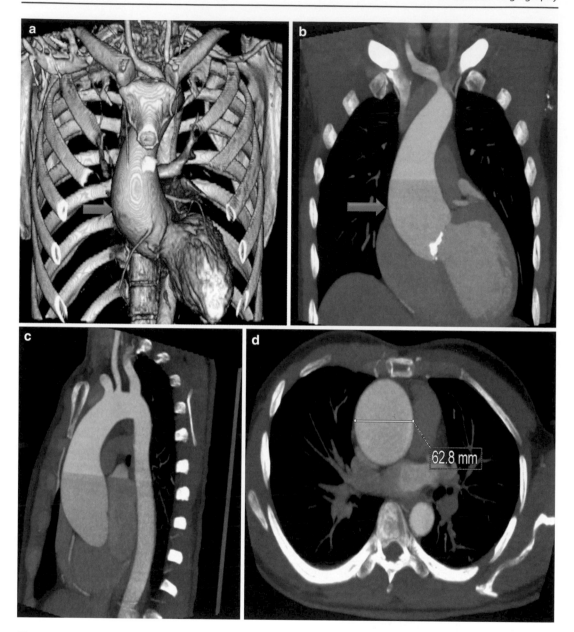

Fig. 8.4 3D volume rendered (**a**), coronal maximum intensity projection (**b**), sagittal maximum intensity projection (**c**), and axial (**d**) reconstructions demonstrating fusiform dilatation of the ascending aorta (*blue arrow*). *Ascending aortic diameter is normally up to 3.5 cm, with increasing risk of rupture with increasing size and/or rate of growth*

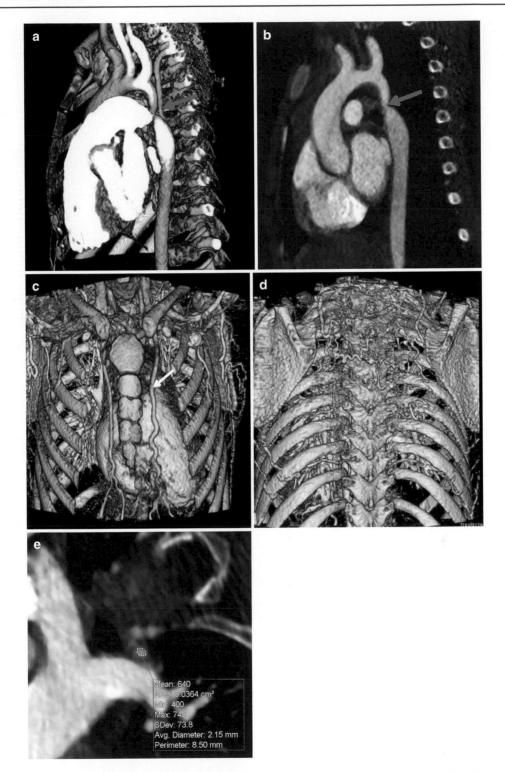

Fig. 8.5 3D volume rendered (**a**, **c**, **d**) and sagittal (**b**) reconstructions, with semi-automated vessel analysis (**e**), demonstrating extensive collateralization and associated enlargement of the left internal mammary artery (*white arrow*) (**c**). Post-stenotic dilatation of the decending aorta gives the characteristic "figure 3" appearance on sagittal view (**a**, **b**), with focal narrowing centrally (*blue arrow*). *Vessel analysis* (**e**) *allows quantification of the degree of stenosis, which differentiates this entity from pseudocoarctation, wherein there is elongation and buckling of the aorta without hemodynamic compromise*

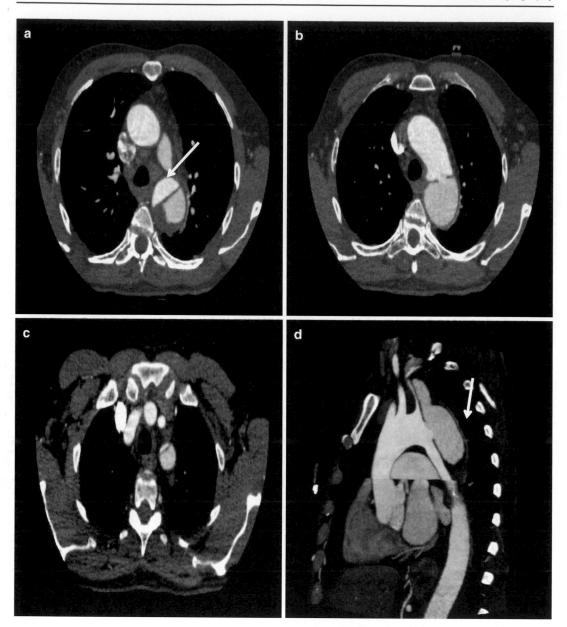

Fig. 8.6 Axial (**a–c**) and sagittal (**d**) reconstructions depicting a proximal descending aortic dissection (*white arrow*), with extension into the left common carotid artery. The intimal flap is easily identified, delineating true from false lumen. Here the true lumen is more intensely contrast-opacified, as is the usual case. Within the dependent portion of the false lumen, a filling defect compatible with thrombus is also identified (*white arrows*) (**a, c**)

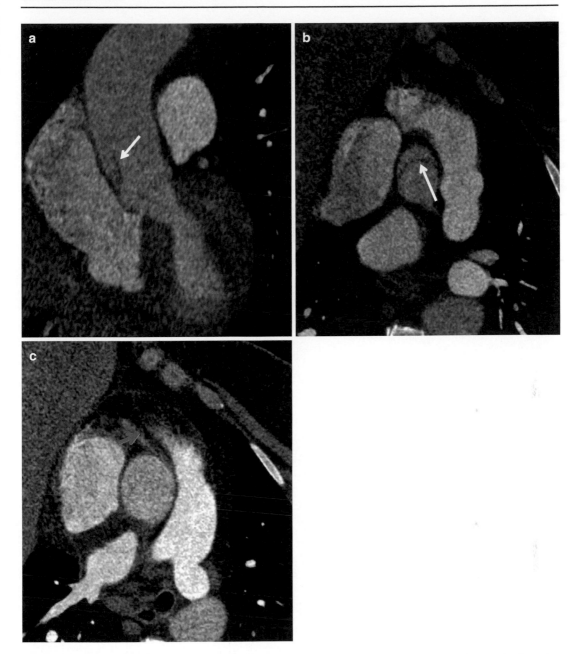

Fig. 8.7 Oblique sagittal (**a**) and oblique axial (**b**, **c**) reconstructions demonstrating a type A aortic dissection with involvement of the root. Multiple views are necessary to confirm the luminal flap versus valve leaflet (*white arrows*). Poor contrast filling (**c**) of the right coronary artery (*blue arrow*) suggests obstruction by the dissecting flap. *This is a surgical emergency, emphasizing the importance of identifying the origins of the coronary arteries in the presence of dissection*

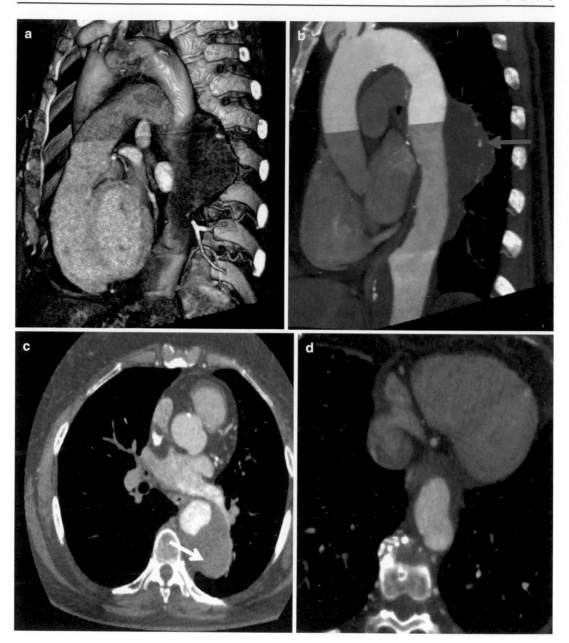

Fig. 8.8 3D volume rendered (**a**), sagittal maximum intensity projection (**b**), and axial (**c, d**) reconstructions illustrating a chronic type B aortic dissection. Chronicity is determined after 14 days. As medical management is the mainstay of most type B dissection, these are primarily the subtypes of dissection that are followed by serial imaging. Note the luminal remodeling (**c**) and complete thrombosis of the false lumen (*white arrow*), whose outer margin (**b**) is delineated by residual calcified atherosclerotic plaque (*blue arrow*)

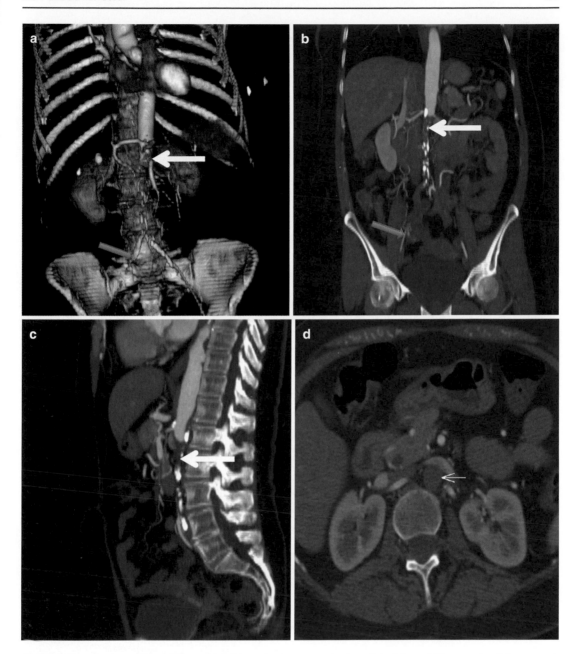

Fig. 8.9 3D volume rendered (**a**), coronal (**b**), sagittal maximum intensity projection (**c**), and axial (**d**) reconstructions demonstrating complete occlusion of the infrarenal aorta. No contrast is seen within the aorta (**b**) below the origins of the renal arteries (*white arrow*). Distal reconstitution of the bilateral iliac arteries (*blue arrows*) (**d**) can occur via multiple potential collateral routes, in this case via superior-to-inferior epigastric arteries. Presence of collaterals is compatible with chronic progressive occlusion

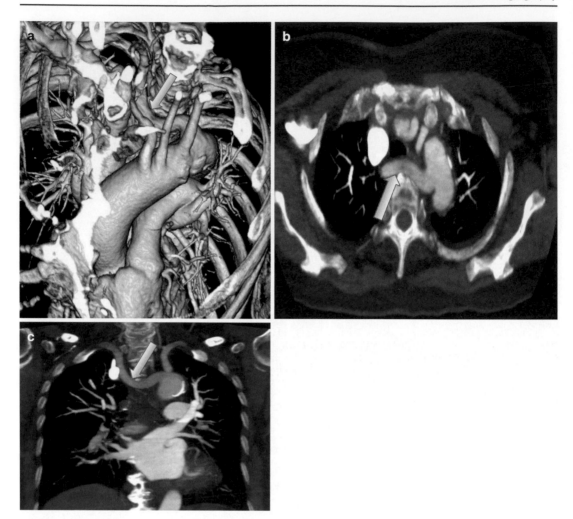

Fig. 8.10 3D volume rendered (**a**), axial maximum intensity projection (**b**), and coronal maximum intensity projection (**c**) reconstructions demonstrating the dilated origin of an aberrant retroesophageal right subclavian artery (*white arrows*) (**a**, **b**). This is usually an isolated finding, and may rarely be symptomatic from esophageal compression. This is a mirror image of the classically described Kommerell's diverticulum, the dilated origin of an aberrant left subclavian in association with a right-sided aortic arch. These may be associated with symptomatic airway or esophageal compression

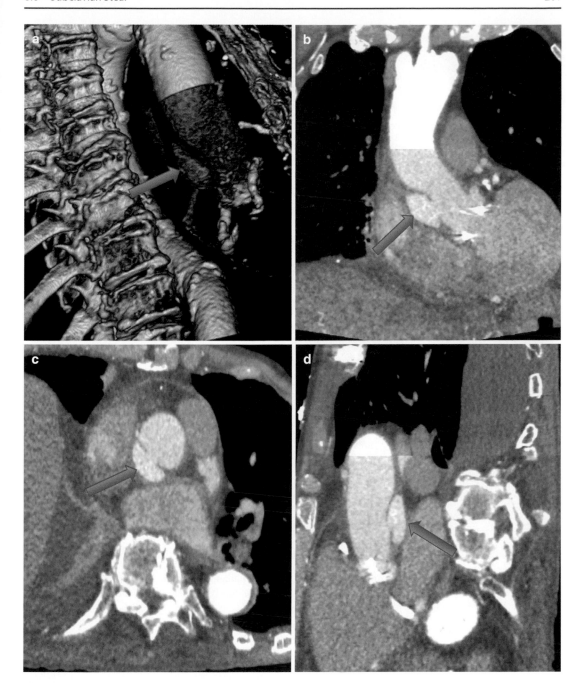

Fig. 8.11 3D volume rendered (**a**), coronal (**b**), axial (**c**), and oblique sagittal (**d**) reconstructions demonstrating a focal contrast-filled outpouching from the aortic root (*blue arrow*). Leaking pseudoaneurysms such as this typi-cally result from traumatic deceleration injury, commonly involving the aortic isthmus (95 %); rarely the aortic root, as in this case

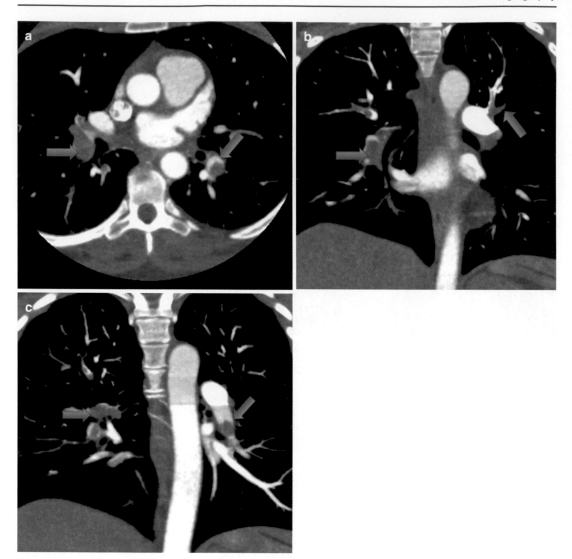

Fig. 8.12 Axial (**a**), and coronal (**b**, **c**) reconstructions demonstrating large filling defects in multiple pulmonary artery branches bilaterally (*blue arrow*), compatible with bilateral pulmonary emboli. The extensive clot burden in this case involves lobar, segmental, and subsegmental branches

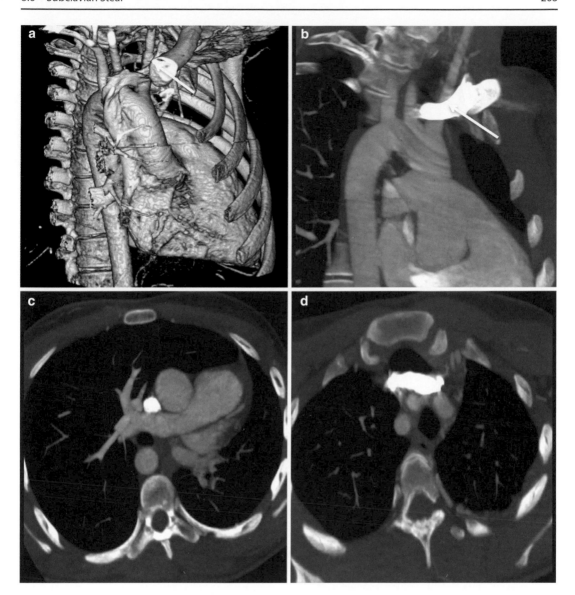

Fig. 8.13 3D volume rendered (**a**), oblique coronal maximum intensity projection (**b**), and axial maximum intensity projections (**c**, **d**) demonstrating a right-sided aortic arch. *Retrotracheal and retroesophageal inspection reveals absence of an aberrant vessel, which can be asso-ciated.* Note the arch origin of the right subclavian artery and presence of left brachiocephalic artery (*white arrows*), compatible with mirror image branch pattern of the great vessels. This configuration is associated with cyanotic congenital heart disease

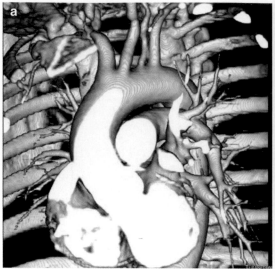 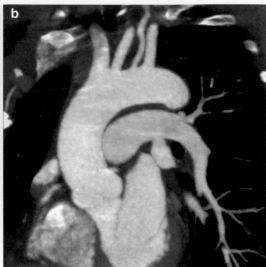

Fig. 8.14 3D volume rendered (**a**) and oblique coronal maximum intensity projection (**b**) reconstructions demonstrating anomalous origin of the left vertebral artery directly from the aortic arch. This variant configuration is seen in approximately 10 % of the population. Normally, the left vertebral arises from the left subclavian artery

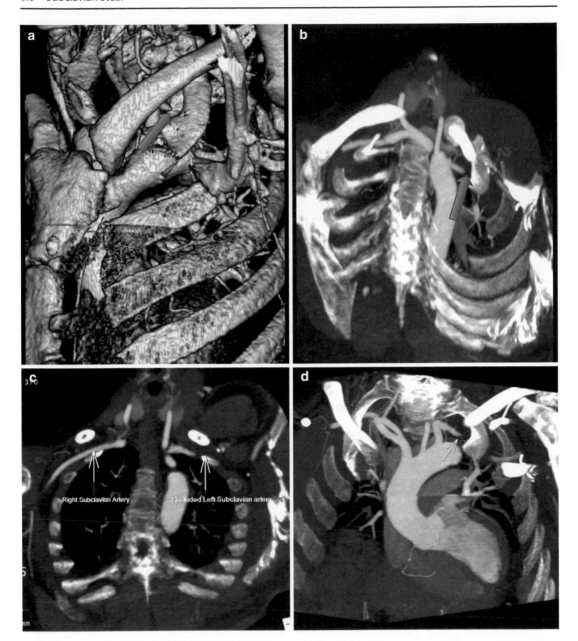

Fig. 8.15 3D volume rendered (**a**), oblique axial (**b, c**) and coronal (**d**) maximum intensity projection reconstructions demonstrating an abrupt filling defect within the left subclavian artery (*blue arrow*) during its course between the clavicle and first rib (*white arrow*)

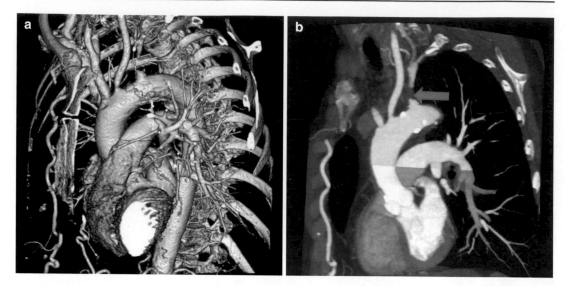

Fig. 8.16 3D volume rendered (**a**) and oblique sagittal maximum intensity projection (**b**) reconstructions demonstrating an abrupt filling defect within the proximal left subclavian artery (*blue arrow*). This type of occlusion has myriad causes, and care should be taken to identify the origins of the major branch vessels including vertebral artery. Distal reconstitution may result from collateralization or, if the occlusion is very proximal, retrograde vertebral artery flow

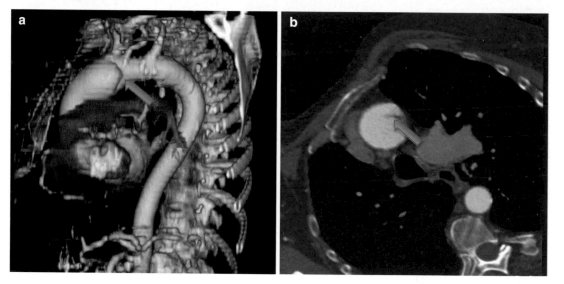

Fig. 8.17 3D volume rendered (**a**), oblique axial maximum intensity projection (**b**) reconstructions demonstrating outpouching of the ascending aorta with associated luminal flap, compatible with a penetrating ulcer (*blue arrow*). This is distinguished from an ulcerated plaque by its extension beyond the aortic wall, and can be thought of as a continuation of the same atherosclerotic process. A variable degree of dissection can be associated, which can progress to true dissection when the luminal flap extends across the aorta, creating true and false lumen

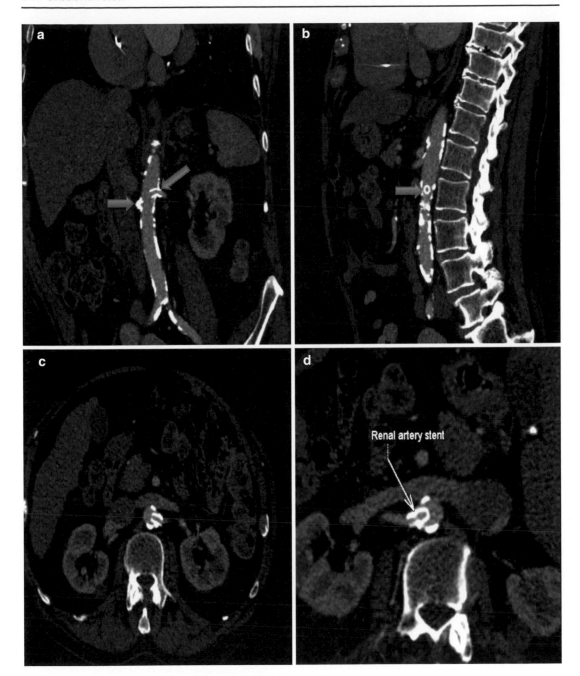

Fig. 8.18 Coronal (**a**), sagittal (**b**) reconstructions demonstrating bilateral renal artery stents (*blue arrows*). Axial (**c**, **d**) reconstructions demonstrating protrusion of the left renal artery stent in the lumen of the abdominal aorta (*white arrow*). Continuity with relative uniformity of the parallel stent walls helps distinguish it from calcification

References

1. Bickerstaff LK, Pairolero PC, Hollier LH, et al. Thoracic aortic aneurysms: a population-based study. Surgery. 1982;92:1103.
2. Graham M, Chan A. Ultrasound screening for clinically occult abdominal aortic aneurysm. CMAJ. 1988;138:627.
3. Scott RA, Ashton HA, Kay DN. Abdominal aortic aneurysm in 4237 screened patients: prevalence, development and management over 6 years. Br J Surg. 1991;78:1122.
4. Lederle FA, Johnson GR, Wilson SE, et al. Prevalence and associations of abdominal aortic aneurysm detected through screening. Aneurysm Detection and Management (ADAM) Veterans Affairs Cooperative Study Group. Ann Intern Med. 1997;126:441.
5. Larsson E, Vishnevskaya L, Kalin B, et al. High frequency of thoracic aneurysms in patients with abdominal aortic aneurysms. Ann Surg. 2011;253:180.
6. Larson EW, Edwards WD. Risk factors for aortic dissection: a necropsy study of 161 cases. Am J Cardiol. 1984;53:849.
7. Clouse WD, Hallett Jr JW, Schaff HV, et al. Acute aortic dissection: population-based incidence compared with degenerative aortic aneurysm rupture. Mayo Clin Proc. 2004;79:176.
8. Hagan PG, Nienaber CA, Isselbacher EM, et al. The International Registry of Acute Aortic Dissection (IRAD): new insights into an old disease. JAMA. 2000;283:897.
9. Reller MD, Strickland MJ, Riehle-Colarusso T, et al. Prevalence of congenital heart defects in metropolitan Atlanta, 1998–2005. J Pediatr. 2008;153:807.
10. Hoffman JI, Kaplan S. The incidence of congenital heart disease. J Am Coll Cardiol. 2002;39:1890.
11. Gentile R, Stevenson G, Dooley T, et al. Pulsed Doppler echocardiographic determination of time of ductal closure in normal newborn infants. J Pediatr. 1981;98:443.
12. Davidson HR. A large family with patent ductus arteriosus and unusual face. J Med Genet. 1993;30:503.
13. Horlander KT, Mannino DM, Leeper KV. Pulmonary embolism mortality in the United States, 1979–1998: an analysis using multiple-cause mortality data. Arch Intern Med. 2003;163:1711.
14. Kröger K, Küpper-Nybelen J, Moerchel C, et al. Prevalence and economic burden of pulmonary embolism in Germany. Vasc Med. 2012;17:303.
15. Wiener RS, Schwartz LM, Woloshin S. Time trends in pulmonary embolism in the United States: evidence of overdiagnosis. Arch Intern Med. 2011;171:831.
16. Bornstein NM, Norris JW. Subclavian steal: a harmless haemodynamic phenomenon? Lancet. 1986;2:303.
17. Hennerici M, Klemm C, Rautenberg W. The subclavian steal phenomenon: a common vascular disorder with rare neurologic deficits. Neurology. 1988;38:669.
18. Labropoulos N, Nandivada P, Berkelis K. Prevalence and impact of the subclavian steal. Ann Surg. 2010;252(1):166–70.

Incidental Findings in Cardiac CTA

9

Rajesh Gupta and Muhammad A. Musani

Coronary artery CT evaluation is now widely performed on MDCT scanners with protocols optimized for high spatial resolution and reconstruction in various planes and fields of view [1]. Additionally, techniques may utilize contrast and thinner slice selection. This presents an opportunity to visualize and analyze other organs and structures besides the heart. Most commonly, the lungs, mediastinum, pulmonary vasculature, diaphragm, upper abdomen, and osseous as well as soft tissue structures of the thorax can be included in the field of view [2]. There has been a surge of reported extracardiac incidental findings that are discovered on coronary CT examinations and acknowledging them may be necessary as some are clinically significant and may require immediate action versus follow-up recommendations [3].

There is controversy surrounding the reporting of extracardiac incidental findings discovered on routine coronary CT protocols. Opponents argue that these incidental findings may lead to further investigations that would result in inappropriate resource utilization, increased healthcare costs, and increased patient anxiety [2]. Supporters argue that all data should be collected and if additional findings are indeterminate or significant, the physician has an ethical duty to act in the patient's best interest [3].

Several technical factors will increase the prevalence of identifying incidental findings on routine interpretation of a coronary CT. The use of 64-slice MDCT coronary CTA, thinner slices, and advanced reconstruction algorithms provides superior spatial and temporal resolution and anatomic detail allowing for increased detection of incidental findings [4]. Another major contributing factor is the field of view. Volume analysis reveals that 35.5 % of the total chest volume is displayed when MDCT focuses on the heart as opposed to 70.3 % of the chest being visible when raw data is reconstructed with the maximum field of view [1].

Patient selection is another important consideration in regards to the probability of identifying significant incidental findings. Patients undergoing evaluation for coronary disease often times have risk factors and comorbidities that contribute to incidental findings, most commonly in the lungs. It has been reported that there is a significant correlation between any history of smoking and increasing age with the detection of extracardiac incidental findings which leads to imaging follow-up [5]. Given this correlation, it has been suggested that the entire chest be scanned on coronary MDCT for smokers older than 50 years, which may only add an additional 1 mSv of radiation. Interestingly, a statistically significant correlation has not been found between coronary calcium scores, age, and the detection of incidental findings [5]. Presenting symptoms may also increase the likelihood of incidental findings as a patient presenting with undifferentiated acute chest pain or shortness of breath may have extracardiac findings associated with their symptoms like aortic dissection or pulmonary embolism [6].

M.H. Musani et al., *Clinical Pearls in Diagnostic Cardiac Computed Tomographic Angiography*,
DOI 10.1007/978-3-319-08168-7_9, © Springer International Publishing Switzerland 2015

It has been reported that the incidence of incidental findings is 8 % in asymptomatic patients undergoing noncontrast chest CT for coronary artery calcium detection. Alternatively, the incidence may be as high as 58 % in patients with known or suspected coronary artery disease who receive a cardiac CTA, with up to 22 % requiring follow-up investigations [6]. The physician interpreting a cardiac CT must be familiar with potential incidental findings that can be encountered in order to identify them. Additionally, a determination must be made on whether a finding is benign, indeterminate, or significant. Then based on provided history and access to prior examinations, the physician must decide whether to report a certain finding and if follow-up investigations need to be recommended.

The most common extracardiac incidental finding reported during a cardiac CT evaluation is a pulmonary nodule. Recommendations for follow-up imaging of incidental solid (noncalcified) pulmonary nodules are usually based on established Fleischner Society guidelines [6]. Modified follow-up recommendation methodology has been proposed on cardiac CT, a 1-year follow-up examination for noncalcified nodules 2–5 mm in size, 6-month follow-up for nodules 6–9 mm in size, and immediate follow-up imaging for nodules larger than 9 mm [7].

Clinically significant pulmonary incidental findings that require immediate follow-up include noncalcified nodules greater than 9 mm to 1.0 cm in size and lung masses, defined as size greater than 3.0 cm. Figure 9.1 shows a lung mass that is very concerning for cancer as it erodes the anterior left rib. There have been several cases of patients with shortness of breath undergoing coronary CTA who are found to have multiple pulmonary emboli, which often requires immediate attention [8]. Incidental discovery of pneumonia is critical to report. Figure 9.2 demonstrates a case of bilateral lower lobe pneumonia which follow-up to resolution imaging in 6–8 weeks post therapy should be recommended. Identification of a pneumothorax is extremely important, especially if the patient is undergoing cardiac CTA evaluation for chest pain, which will likely require changing of imaging protocols and initial management depending on size and complications [6].

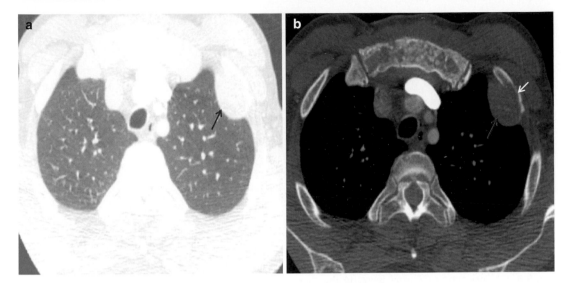

Fig. 9.1 (a) Postcontrast CT axial image of the chest shows an extrapleural soft tissue mass in the anterior left upper chest measuring up to 4.0 cm in lung windows (*red arrow*) (b). Bone windows show the mass eroding the anterior left rib (*white arrow*). This mass is consistent with an aggressive lung cancer destroying the adjacent bone. The patient presented with chest pain. Follow-up recommendations included a complete contrast-enhanced chest, abdomen, and pelvis and possible CT-guided biopsy

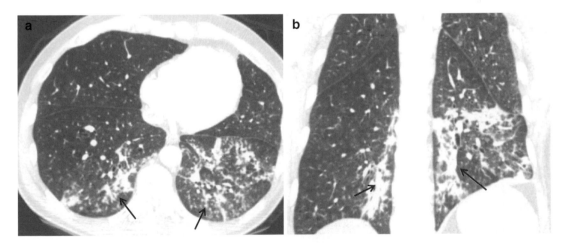

Fig. 9.2 (a) Postcontrast CT image in lung windows displays dense consolidation in the left lower lobe and right lower lobe (*red arrows*) consistent with pneumonia. (b) Coronal reformatted image in lung windows again identifies bilateral lower lobe pneumonia (*red arrows*). Follow-up imaging to confirm resolution should be recommended

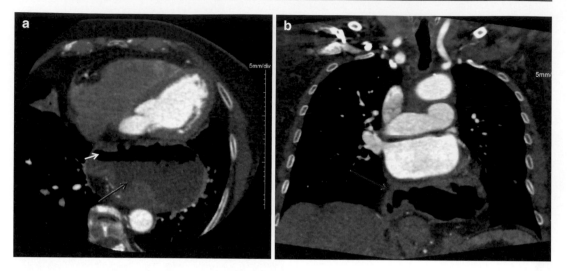

Fig. 9.3 (a) Postcontrast CT axial image of the chest shows a 5.3×7.6 cm soft tissue density posterior to the heart in the region of the esophagus (*red arrow*) containing air (*white arrow*) which is consistent with a hiatal hernia. (b) A coronal reformatted image again shows the hiatal hernia (*red arrow*). *Most hiatal hernias are of the sliding type where the GE junction and sometimes gastric fundus is displaced above the esophageal hiatus.* The patient was asymptomatic and undergoing preoperative evaluation, and so this is a benign finding that does not require follow-up. However, if a large portion of the stomach is displaced, there is risk for volvulus, obstruction, and ischemia that may require surgery

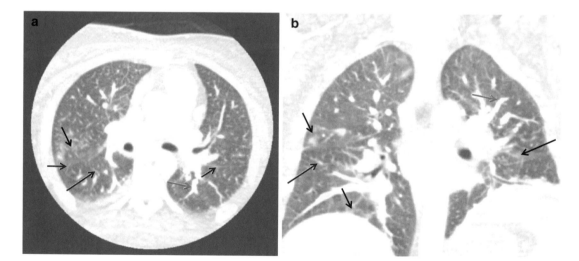

Fig. 9.4 (a) Postcontrast axial image demonstrates diffuse severe interlobular septal thickening (*red arrows*) and dependent ground-glass opacities (*black arrows*) consistent with pulmonary edema. The pulmonary vasculature is engorged and extends peripherally (*blue arrows*). (b) Coronal reformatted image in lung windows re-demonstrates pulmonary edema with interlobular septal thickening (*red arrow*), ground-glass opacities (*black arrows*), and pulmonary vasculature engorgement (*blue arrow*)". The patient was a 37-year-old female with ESRD on hemodialysis with pleuritic chest pain. The patient should undergo follow-up imaging to confirm resolution after therapy

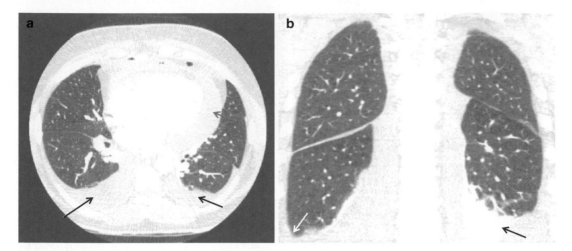

Fig. 9.5 (a) Postcontrast axial CT image in lung windows show bilateral fluid densities in the posterior chest following the pleural contour consistent with moderate sized pleural effusions (*red arrows*). Additionally, this patient has a pericardial effusion (*blue arrow*). (b) Coronal reformatted image again partially shows the pleural effusion (*red arrow*). Another clue is blunting of the costophrenic angles (*white arrows*). Follow-up to confirm resolution may be recommended depending on prior examinations and clinical symptoms

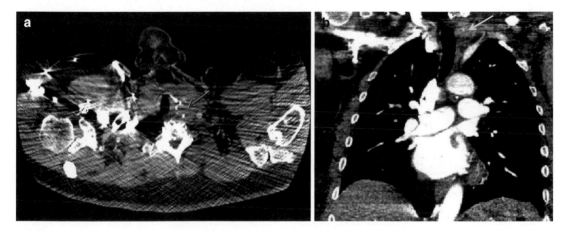

Fig. 9.6 (a) There is a heterogeneously enlarged left thyroid lobe, with internal calcification (*red arrow*). (b) Coronal reformatted image shows that this enlarged thyroid lobe (*yellow arrow*) has intrathoracic extension into the prevascular space (not seen on this image). These findings were stable when compared to prior imaging so no follow-up needed to be recommended. If it were a new finding, additional imaging such as an ultrasound could be suggested

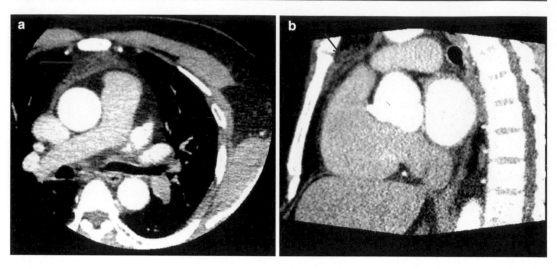

Fig. 9.7 (**a**) Postcontrast 320-slice axial CT image shows anterior mediastinal linear and nodular soft tissue densities within the expected thymic space (*red arrows*). (**b**) These soft tissue densities are again identified on the sagittal reformatted image (*red arrow*). Clinical history correlation is recommended

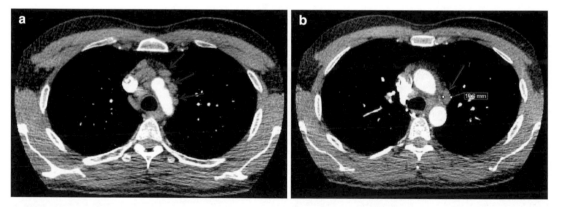

Fig. 9.8 (**a**) Postcontrast 320-slice CT axial image shows multiple prominent and enlarged lymph nodes (*red arrows*). These soft tissue densities do not follow a vascular course which is apparent on postcontrast images. (**b**) Another axial image displays the largest measuring about 11 mm in the short axis (*red arrow*). The patient has a history of sarcoidosis and presented with atypical chest pain. The lymph nodes were stable when compared to prior imaging

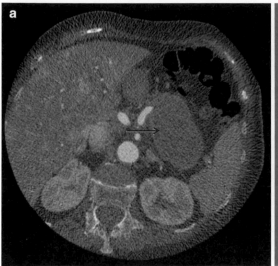
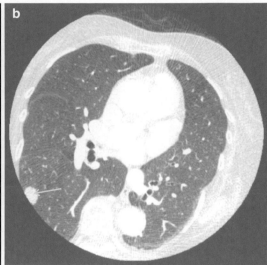

Fig. 9.9 (**a**) Postcontrast CT axial image shows a large pancreatic body mass which was pancreatic cancer (*red arrow*). (**b**) Axial image in lung windows shows an associated lung mass consistent with metastasis (*yellow arrow*). Comparison was made with outside imaging which clearly demonstrated the pancreatic mass. The patient presented with atypical chest pain for a triple rule out

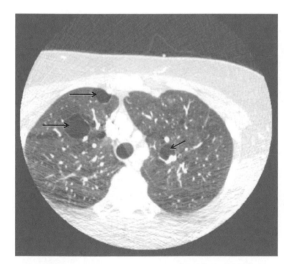

Fig. 9.10 Postcontrast CT axial image in lung windows displays multiple scattered focal airspaces with thin, almost imperceptible walls consistent with pulmonary blebs and bullae (*red arrows*). Pulmonary blebs increase the risk for spontaneous pneumothorax and therefore they should be reported so the clinical team can decide further treatment options

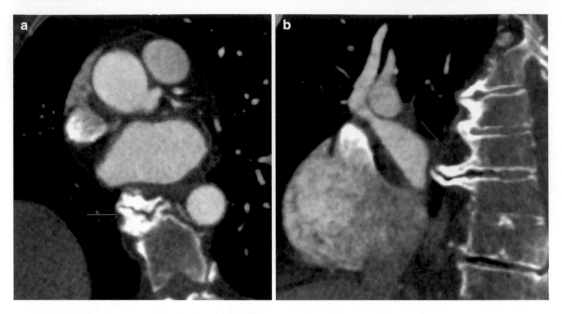

Fig. 9.11 (**a**) Postcontrast CT axial image reveals a large anterior osteophyte complex extending from the vertebral body (*red arrow*). (**b**) Sagittal image demonstrates the large osteophyte (*red arrow*).

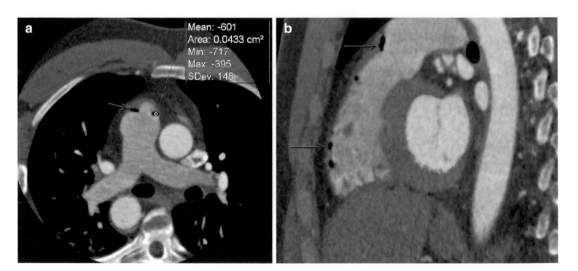

Fig. 9.12 (**a**) Postcontrast CT axial image demonstrates air within the right ventricle (*red arrow*). (**b**) Sagittal image displays further tracking of the air down the anterior surface of the right ventricle (*red arrows*).

References

1. Haller S, Kaiser C, Buser P, et al. Coronary artery imaging with contrast-enhanced MDCT: extracardiac findings. AJR Am J Roentgenol. 2006;187:105–10.
2. MacHaalany J, Yam Y, Ruddy TD, et al. Potential clinical and economic consequences of noncardiac incidental findings on cardiac computed tomography. J Am Coll Cardiol. 2009;54(16):1533–41.
3. Hlatky MA, Iribarren C. The dilemma of incidental findings on cardiac computed tomography. J Am Coll Cardiol. 2009;54:1542–3.
4. Kirsch J, Araoz PA, Steinberg FB, et al. Prevalence and significance of incidental extracardiac findings at 64-multidetector coronary CTA. J Thorac Imaging. 2007;22:330–4.
5. Lee CI, Tsai EB, Sigal BM, et al. Incidental extracardiac findings at coronary CT: clinical and economic impact. AJR Am J Roentgenol. 2010;194:1531–8.
6. Lehman SJ, Abbara S, Cury RC, et al. Significance of cardiac computed tomography incidental findings in acute chest pain. Am J Med. 2009;122:543–9.
7. Burt JR, Iribarren C, Fair JM, et al. Incidental findings on cardiac multidetector row computed tomography among healthy older adults: prevalence and clinical correlates. Arch Intern Med. 2008;168:756–61.
8. Tseng P, Budoff M. Cardiac anatomy by CT. In: Budoff MJ, Shinbane JS, editors. Cardiac CT imaging: diagnosis of cardiovascular disease. London: Springer; 2006. p. 38–9.

Index

Printing and Binding: PHOENIX PRINT GmbH, Würzburg